THE TEACHINGS OF

The
Joshua
Diet
Playbook

VOLUME II

Printed in the United States of America

First Printing, 2016

ISBN-13: 978-1541082489

ISBN: 1541082486

Write five affirmations:

1. ....
2. ....
3. ....
4. ....
5. ....

How did you feel today (or yesterday if you're writing this in the morning)?

....

....

How do you feel now? ....

How do you intend to feel today (or tomorrow if you're writing this in the evening)?

....

....

INSPIRATION:

Did you receive inspiration today (or yesterday if you're writing this in the morning)?

....

....

Describe what you were inspired to do or say ....

....

FOOD EXPERIMENT:

What single item of food did you experiment with today (or yesterday if you're writing this in the morning)? ....

Describe how you felt? ....

....

Does your unique body process this food easily? ....

How did you feel today (or yesterday if you're writing this in the morning)?

....

QUOTE OF THE DAY:

" You are the creator of you and you can create whatever you like. You have the ability to be, do and have everything you want in this reality. The universe yields you your wishes as long as you understand how your point of focus creates your reality." *Joshua*

MEDITATION:

Duration .... Type...

Time of Day .... Satisfaction Level: 1 2 3 4 5 6 7 8 9 10

Notes: ....

....

....

Appreciation: (List 5 things you appreciate about your life)

1. ....

2. ....

3. ....

4. ....

5. ....

Gratitude: (List 5 things you are grateful for, which can include future manifestations)

1. ....

2. ....

3. ....

4. ....

5. ....

Set your general intentions for the day:

....

....

....

....

Write five affirmations:

1. ....

2. ....

3. ....

4. ....

5. ....

How did you feel today (or yesterday if you're writing this in the morning)?

....

....

How do you feel now? ....

How do you intend to feel today (or tomorrow if you're writing this in the evening)?

....

....

INSPIRATION:

Did you receive inspiration today (or yesterday if you're writing this in the morning)?

....

....

Describe what you were inspired to do or say ....

....

FOOD EXPERIMENT:

What single item of food did you experiment with today (or yesterday if you're writing this in the morning)? ....

Describe how you felt? ....

....

Does your unique body process this food easily? ....

How did you feel today (or yesterday if you're writing this in the morning)?

....

QUOTE OF THE DAY:

" You are worthy of living the life you desire. You are a worthy being, as worthy as any who has ever lived. There is not another person on Earth who is more worthy than you. You are worthy enough to love and to be loved. You are worthy enough to have the body you desire. But don't for a moment believe that having a nice body will make you feel worthy. It will not." *Joshua*

MEDITATION:

Duration .... Type..

Time of Day .... Satisfaction Level: 1 2 3 4 5 6 7 8 9 10

Notes: ....

....

Appreciation: (List 5 things you appreciate about your life)

1. ....

2. ....

3. ....

4. ....

5. ....

Gratitude: (List 5 things you are grateful for, which can include future manifestations)

1. ....

2. ....

3. ....

4. ....

5. ....

Set your general intentions for the day:

....

....

....

....

Write five affirmations:

1. ....

2. ....

3. ....

4. ....

5. ....

How did you feel today (or yesterday if you're writing this in the morning)?

....

....

How do you feel now? ....

How do you intend to feel today (or tomorrow if you're writing this in the evening)?

....

....

INSPIRATION:

Did you receive inspiration today (or yesterday if you're writing this in the morning)?

....

....

Describe what you were inspired to do or say ....

....

FOOD EXPERIMENT:

What single item of food did you experiment with today (or yesterday if you're writing this in the morning)? ....

Describe how you felt? ....

....

Does your unique body process this food easily?...

How did you feel today (or yesterday if you're writing this in the morning)?

....

QUOTE OF THE DAY:

" If the fear is irrational, meaning it can't kill you, then it is false. All irrational fears are false. They seem real, but they are not. You can prove that an irrational fear is false. You can find evidence that it is false. When you show yourself evidence that the irrational fear is false, you reduce the intensity of that fear." *Joshua*

MEDITATION:

Duration .... Type..

Time of Day .... Satisfaction Level: 1 2 3 4 5 6 7 8 9 10

Notes: ....

....

....

Appreciation: (List 5 things you appreciate about your life)

1. ....

2. ....

3. ....

4. ....

5. ....

Gratitude: (List 5 things you are grateful for, which can include future manifestations)

1. ....

2. ....

3. ....

4. ....

5. ....

Set your general intentions for the day:

....

....

....

....

Write five affirmations:

1. ....

2. ....

3. ....

4. ....

5. ....

How did you feel today (or yesterday if you're writing this in the morning)?

....

....

How do you feel now? ....

How do you intend to feel today (or tomorrow if you're writing this in the evening)?

....

....

INSPIRATION:

Did you receive inspiration today (or yesterday if you're writing this in the morning)?

....

....

Describe what you were inspired to do or say ....

....

FOOD EXPERIMENT:

What single item of food did you experiment with today (or yesterday if you're writing this in the morning)? ....

Describe how you felt? ....

....

Does your unique body process this food easily?..

How did you feel today (or yesterday if you're writing this in the morning)?

....

QUOTE OF THE DAY:

❝ All thoughts exist in the nonphysical and your vibration attracts the thoughts that resonate with how you're feeling in the moment. Change the way you feel and you change what the universe brings to you. Change your emotional state of being and you change the quality of thoughts that come to you." *Joshua*

MEDITATION:

Duration .... Type...

Time of Day .... Satisfaction Level: 1 2 3 4 5 6 7 8 9 10

Notes: ....

....

....

Appreciation: (List 5 things you appreciate about your life)

1. ....

2. ....

3. ....

4. ....

5. ....

Gratitude: (List 5 things you are grateful for, which can include future manifestations)

1. ....

2. ....

3. ....

4. ....

5. ....

Set your general intentions for the day:

....

....

....

....

Write five affirmations:

1. ....

2. ....

3. ....

4. ....

5. ....

How did you feel today (or yesterday if you're writing this in the morning)?

....

....

How do you feel now? ....

How do you intend to feel today (or tomorrow if you're writing this in the evening)?

....

....

INSPIRATION:

Did you receive inspiration today (or yesterday if you're writing this in the morning)?

....

....

Describe what you were inspired to do or say ....

....

FOOD EXPERIMENT:

What single item of food did you experiment with today (or yesterday if you're writing this in the morning)? ....

Describe how you felt? ....

....

Does your unique body process this food easily? ....

How did you feel today (or yesterday if you're writing this in the morning)?

....

QUOTE OF THE DAY:

" What you believe to be true, is. What you expect, comes. Your thoughts form your reality. This is how physical reality was designed. If you want to change your reality, you simply change your beliefs, expectations, and thoughts." *Joshua*

MEDITATION:

Duration .... Type..

Time of Day .... Satisfaction Level: 1   2   3   4   5   6   7   8   9   10

Notes: ....

....

Appreciation: (List 5 things you appreciate about your life)

1. ....

2. ....

3. ....

4. ....

5. ....

Gratitude: (List 5 things you are grateful for, which can include future manifestations)

1. ....

2. ....

3. ....

4. ....

5. ....

Set your general intentions for the day:

....

....

....

....

....

Write five affirmations:

1. ....

2. ....

3. ....

4. ....

5. ....

How did you feel today (or yesterday if you're writing this in the morning)?

....

....

How do you feel now? ....

How do you intend to feel today (or tomorrow if you're writing this in the evening)?

....

....

INSPIRATION:

Did you receive inspiration today (or yesterday if you're writing this in the morning)?

....

....

Describe what you were inspired to do or say ....

....

FOOD EXPERIMENT:

What single item of food did you experiment with today (or yesterday if you're writing this in the morning)? ....

Describe how you felt? ....

....

Does your unique body process this food easily? ....

How did you feel today (or yesterday if you're writing this in the morning)?

....

QUOTE OF THE DAY:

❝ Limiting beliefs are based in fear and are therefore untrue. Beneficial beliefs are based in love and are therefore true." *Joshua*

MEDITATION:

Duration .... Type...

Time of Day .... Satisfaction Level: 1 2 3 4 5 6 7 8 9 10

Notes: ....

....

....

Appreciation: (List 5 things you appreciate about your life)

1. ....

2. ....

3. ....

4. ....

5. ....

Gratitude: (List 5 things you are grateful for, which can include future manifestations)

1. ....

2. ....

3. ....

4. ....

5. ....

Set your general intentions for the day:

....

....

....

....

Write five affirmations:

1. ....
2. ....
3. ....
4. ....
5. ....

How did you feel today (or yesterday if you're writing this in the morning)?

....

....

How do you feel now? ....

How do you intend to feel today (or tomorrow if you're writing this in the evening)?

....

....

INSPIRATION:

Did you receive inspiration today (or yesterday if you're writing this in the morning)?

....

....

Describe what you were inspired to do or say ....

....

FOOD EXPERIMENT:

What single item of food did you experiment with today (or yesterday if you're writing this in the morning)? ....

Describe how you felt? ....

....

Does your unique body process this food easily? ....

How did you feel today (or yesterday if you're writing this in the morning)?

....

DAY 10: _____ / _____ / _____   M T W T F S S

QUOTE OF THE DAY:

" You must realize that you are unique and you came to this reality to explore Earth in your own unique way. You chose your body for this mission. It is an important part of your trajectory. Your body is your space suit. It was specifically designed for you based on the life you intended to live prior to your birth. Your height, sex, weight, skin color, and shape were all intended to give you the best possibility to explore the life you wanted to explore. It was a decision made with great care and thought." *Joshua*

MEDITATION:

Duration .... Type..

Time of Day .... Satisfaction Level: 1 2 3 4 5 6 7 8 9 10

Notes: ....

....

Appreciation: (List 5 things you appreciate about your life)

1. ....

2. ....

3. ....

4. ....

5. ....

Gratitude: (List 5 things you are grateful for, which can include future manifestations)

1. ....

2. ....

3. ....

4. ....

5. ....

Set your general intentions for the day:

....

....

....

Write five affirmations:

1. ....
2. ....
3. ....
4. ....
5. ....

How did you feel today (or yesterday if you're writing this in the morning)?

....

....

How do you feel now? ....

How do you intend to feel today (or tomorrow if you're writing this in the evening)?

....

....

INSPIRATION:

Did you receive inspiration today (or yesterday if you're writing this in the morning)?

....

....

Describe what you were inspired to do or say ....

....

FOOD EXPERIMENT:

What single item of food did you experiment with today (or yesterday if you're writing this in the morning)? ....

Describe how you felt? ....

....

Does your unique body process this food easily? ....

How did you feel today (or yesterday if you're writing this in the morning)?

....

QUOTE OF THE DAY:

❝ When you ignore a negative emotion and resist the situation by calling it wrong or bad, you cause inner conflict and stress on the body. When you refuse to see it from another perspective or find evidence to prove it's false, you cause more stress because you're resisting the message." *Joshua*

MEDITATION:

Duration .... Type...

Time of Day .... Satisfaction Level: 1 2 3 4 5 6 7 8 9 10

Notes: ....

....

....

Appreciation: (List 5 things you appreciate about your life)

1. ....

2. ....

3. ....

4. ....

5. ....

Gratitude: (List 5 things you are grateful for, which can include future manifestations)

1. ....

2. ....

3. ....

4. ....

5. ....

Set your general intentions for the day:

....

....

....

....

Write five affirmations:

1. ....
2. ....
3. ....
4. ....
5. ....

How did you feel today (or yesterday if you're writing this in the morning)?

....

....

How do you feel now? ....

How do you intend to feel today (or tomorrow if you're writing this in the evening)?

....

....

INSPIRATION:

Did you receive inspiration today (or yesterday if you're writing this in the morning)?

....

....

Describe what you were inspired to do or say ....

....

FOOD EXPERIMENT:

What single item of food did you experiment with today (or yesterday if you're writing this in the morning)? ....

Describe how you felt? ....

....

Does your unique body process this food easily? ....

How did you feel today (or yesterday if you're writing this in the morning)?

....

QUOTE OF THE DAY:

66 Focus is the mental practice of keeping your thoughts in alignment with your desire. The power of the mind is an awesome thing to behold. Focus brings the full energy of the mind onto the subject of your attention. When aligned with what you really want and who you really are, the mind engages and leverages universal forces." *Joshua*

MEDITATION:

Duration .... Type..

Time of Day .... Satisfaction Level: 1 2 3 4 5 6 7 8 9 10

Notes: ....

....

Appreciation: (List 5 things you appreciate about your life)

1. ....

2. ....

3. ....

4. ....

5. ....

Gratitude: (List 5 things you are grateful for, which can include future manifestations)

1. ....

2. ....

3. ....

4. ....

5. ....

Set your general intentions for the day:

....

....

....

....

Write five affirmations:

1. ....

2. ....

3. ....

4. ....

5. ....

How did you feel today (or yesterday if you're writing this in the morning)?

....

....

How do you feel now? ....

How do you intend to feel today (or tomorrow if you're writing this in the evening)?

....

....

INSPIRATION:

Did you receive inspiration today (or yesterday if you're writing this in the morning)?

....

....

Describe what you were inspired to do or say ....

....

FOOD EXPERIMENT:

What single item of food did you experiment with today (or yesterday if you're writing this in the morning)? ....

Describe how you felt? ....

....

Does your unique body process this food easily? ....

How did you feel today (or yesterday if you're writing this in the morning)?

....

QUOTE OF THE DAY:

" If you can birth a desire, you can achieve that desire. There's nothing more to it than that. Once you've birthed the desire, you either allow it to come to you or resist it. Once you birth a desire, the universe finds a way to bring it to you. If you allow it to come, by going with the flow and not fighting against things, it will come. If you are constantly arguing with the conditions, you are resisting what you want." *Joshua*

MEDITATION:

Duration .... Type...

Time of Day .... Satisfaction Level: 1 2 3 4 5 6 7 8 9 10

Notes: ....

....

Appreciation: (List 5 things you appreciate about your life)

1. ....

2. ....

3. ....

4. ....

5. ....

Gratitude: (List 5 things you are grateful for, which can include future manifestations)

1. ....

2. ....

3. ....

4. ....

5. ....

Set your general intentions for the day:

....

....

....

Write five affirmations:

1. ....
2. ....
3. ....
4. ....
5. ....

How did you feel today (or yesterday if you're writing this in the morning)?

....

....

How do you feel now? ....

How do you intend to feel today (or tomorrow if you're writing this in the evening)?

....

....

INSPIRATION:

Did you receive inspiration today (or yesterday if you're writing this in the morning)?

....

....

Describe what you were inspired to do or say ....

....

FOOD EXPERIMENT:

What single item of food did you experiment with today (or yesterday if you're writing this in the morning)? ....

Describe how you felt? ....

....

Does your unique body process this food easily? ....

How did you feel today (or yesterday if you're writing this in the morning)?

....

QUOTE OF THE DAY:

" In physical reality, your path is one of moving from a fear-based being to a love-based being. You are in the process of moving from fear to love. You have done this many, many times in countless other lives. In this life, you are closer to being who you really are than in any other life. It is a progression from one life to the next. You are becoming more conscious and self-aware. Everyone is on the journey to becoming who they really are. Some are fighting it and others are progressing with ease and joy." *Joshua*

MEDITATION:

Duration .... Type..

Time of Day .... Satisfaction Level: 1 2 3 4 5 6 7 8 9 10

Notes: ....

....

Appreciation: (List 5 things you appreciate about your life)

1. ....

2. ....

3. ....

4. ....

5. ....

Gratitude: (List 5 things you are grateful for, which can include future manifestations)

1. ....

2. ....

3. ....

4. ....

5. ....

Set your general intentions for the day:

....

....

....

Write five affirmations:

1. ....

2. ....

3. ....

4. ....

5. ....

How did you feel today (or yesterday if you're writing this in the morning)?

....

....

How do you feel now? ....

How do you intend to feel today (or tomorrow if you're writing this in the evening)?

....

....

INSPIRATION:

Did you receive inspiration today (or yesterday if you're writing this in the morning)?

....

....

Describe what you were inspired to do or say ....

....

FOOD EXPERIMENT:

What single item of food did you experiment with today (or yesterday if you're writing this in the morning)? ....

Describe how you felt? ....

....

Does your unique body process this food easily? ....

How did you feel today (or yesterday if you're writing this in the morning)?

....

QUOTE OF THE DAY:

" You are not your persona. You are not really who you think you are. You are far more than that. You have far more to offer. You are far more powerful than you think. You are as worthy as any who have ever lived and you have the ability to access infinite intelligence and leverage the powers of the universe in any way you see fit. You are the creator of your life and you can adopt complete control over the quality of your life. You are responsible for everything in your reality. There is no fate or luck; it is all created by you. You have all the power." *Joshua*

MEDITATION:

Duration .... Type...

Time of Day .... Satisfaction Level: 1 2 3 4 5 6 7 8 9 10

Notes: ....

....

Appreciation: (List 5 things you appreciate about your life)

1. ....

2. ....

3. ....

4. ....

5. ....

Gratitude: (List 5 things you are grateful for, which can include future manifestations)

1. ....

2. ....

3. ....

4. ....

5. ....

Set your general intentions for the day:

....

....

....

Write five affirmations:

1. ....

2. ....

3. ....

4. ....

5. ....

How did you feel today (or yesterday if you're writing this in the morning)?

....

....

How do you feel now? ....

How do you intend to feel today (or tomorrow if you're writing this in the evening)?

....

....

INSPIRATION:

Did you receive inspiration today (or yesterday if you're writing this in the morning)?

....

....

Describe what you were inspired to do or say ....

....

FOOD EXPERIMENT:

What single item of food did you experiment with today (or yesterday if you're writing this in the morning)? ....

Describe how you felt? ....

....

Does your unique body process this food easily? ....

How did you feel today (or yesterday if you're writing this in the morning)?

....

QUOTE OF THE DAY:

" You are the perfect representation of your vibration just as you are. You stand at the perfect place to embark on a new path toward a new desire, just as you are. Your entire life has led up to this moment in time. If you are reading this now, you have reached a vibrational level high enough to resonate with this material. If you want to change the shape of your body, you have lived a life that has unfolded perfectly to create this desire and you have the ability to see it through to its ultimate manifestation." *Joshua*

MEDITATION:

Duration .... Type...

Time of Day .... Satisfaction Level: 1 2 3 4 5 6 7 8 9 10

Notes: ....

....

Appreciation: (List 5 things you appreciate about your life)

1. ....

2. ....

3. ....

4. ....

5. ....

Gratitude: (List 5 things you are grateful for, which can include future manifestations)

1. ....

2. ....

3. ....

4. ....

5. ....

Set your general intentions for the day:

....

....

....

Write five affirmations:

1. ....

2. ....

3. ....

4. ....

5. ....

How did you feel today (or yesterday if you're writing this in the morning)?

....

....

How do you feel now? ....

How do you intend to feel today (or tomorrow if you're writing this in the evening)?

....

....

INSPIRATION:

Did you receive inspiration today (or yesterday if you're writing this in the morning)?

....

....

Describe what you were inspired to do or say ....

....

FOOD EXPERIMENT:

What single item of food did you experiment with today (or yesterday if you're writing this in the morning)? ....

Describe how you felt? ....

....

Does your unique body process this food easily? ....

How did you feel today (or yesterday if you're writing this in the morning)?

....

QUOTE OF THE DAY:

" This is an attractive universe. Everything comes to you. Everything is neutral. You choose what comes by paying attention to it. You decide what is good or bad by your choice of perspective. If you choose a limited perspective, you will see how wrong something is. However, when you choose to look at something from the higher perspective, you are choosing to see that it is not wrong after all. This is the approach to life that will create an atmosphere of allowing. When you are in the state of allowing (not doing), everything you want will begin to flow to you." *Joshua*

MEDITATION:

Duration .... Type...

Time of Day .... Satisfaction Level: 1 2 3 4 5 6 7 8 9 10

Notes: ....

....

Appreciation: (List 5 things you appreciate about your life)

1. ....

2. ....

3. ....

4. ....

5. ....

Gratitude: (List 5 things you are grateful for, which can include future manifestations)

1. ....

2. ....

3. ....

4. ....

5. ....

Set your general intentions for the day:

....

....

....

Write five affirmations:

1. ....

2. ....

3. ....

4. ....

5. ....

How did you feel today (or yesterday if you're writing this in the morning)?

....

....

How do you feel now? ....

How do you intend to feel today (or tomorrow if you're writing this in the evening)?

....

....

INSPIRATION:

Did you receive inspiration today (or yesterday if you're writing this in the morning)?

....

....

Describe what you were inspired to do or say ....

....

FOOD EXPERIMENT:

What single item of food did you experiment with today (or yesterday if you're writing this in the morning)? ....

Describe how you felt? ....

....

Does your unique body process this food easily?...

How did you feel today (or yesterday if you're writing this in the morning)?

....

QUOTE OF THE DAY:

" There is no wrong anywhere in the universe. Anything you perceive to be wrong is simply an illusion created by your limited perspective. Choose the higher perspective and you will see it is right. Everything is right. If you can understand that there is no wrong, that everything is right, and that you have a choice over which perspective you think is more empowering for you, then you will have chosen an approach to life that serves you." *Joshua*

MEDITATION:

Duration .... Type...

Time of Day .... Satisfaction Level: 1 2 3 4 5 6 7 8 9 10

Notes: ....

....

....

Appreciation: (List 5 things you appreciate about your life)

1. ....

2. ....

3. ....

4. ....

5. ....

Gratitude: (List 5 things you are grateful for, which can include future manifestations)

1. ....

2. ....

3. ....

4. ....

5. ....

Set your general intentions for the day:

....

....

....

Write five affirmations:

1. ....

2. ....

3. ....

4. ....

5. ....

How did you feel today (or yesterday if you're writing this in the morning)?

....

....

How do you feel now? ....

How do you intend to feel today (or tomorrow if you're writing this in the evening)?

....

....

INSPIRATION:

Did you receive inspiration today (or yesterday if you're writing this in the morning)?

....

....

Describe what you were inspired to do or say ....

....

FOOD EXPERIMENT:

What single item of food did you experiment with today (or yesterday if you're writing this in the morning)? ....

Describe how you felt? ....

....

Does your unique body process this food easily? ....

How did you feel today (or yesterday if you're writing this in the morning)?

....

QUOTE OF THE DAY:

" Is an emotion physical or nonphysical? It's nonphysical. It has no mass or physical properties. It's like a thought or any other feeling. It exists in the physical world, but can only be felt by the person experiencing the emotion. When you feel fear, others may sense it, but no one knows really what you're experiencing. It is an individual thing. Some people feel fear intensely and others feel it less so. This is true of all emotions." *Joshua*

MEDITATION:

Duration .... Type...

Time of Day .... Satisfaction Level: 1 2 3 4 5 6 7 8 9 10

Notes: ....

....

Appreciation: (List 5 things you appreciate about your life)

1. ....

2. ....

3. ....

4. ....

5. ....

Gratitude: (List 5 things you are grateful for, which can include future manifestations)

1. ....

2. ....

3. ....

4. ....

5. ....

Set your general intentions for the day:

....

....

....

Write five affirmations:

1. ....

2. ....

3. ....

4. ....

5. ....

How did you feel today (or yesterday if you're writing this in the morning)?

....

....

How do you feel now? ....

How do you intend to feel today (or tomorrow if you're writing this in the evening)?

....

....

INSPIRATION:

Did you receive inspiration today (or yesterday if you're writing this in the morning)?

....

....

Describe what you were inspired to do or say ....

....

FOOD EXPERIMENT:

What single item of food did you experiment with today (or yesterday if you're writing this in the morning)? ....

Describe how you felt? ....

....

Does your unique body process this food easily? ....

How did you feel today (or yesterday if you're writing this in the morning)?

....

QUOTE OF THE DAY:

66 If you choose a perspective that does not serve you, you will feel negative emotion every time. Isn't that an excellent system? It never fails. You might choose to ignore the emotion, but it will always be there, every single time. You cannot escape it, thank God. You can't turn it off. It is always on. Even in your dream state. It never fails you. Never ever. It's fail-safe." *Joshua*

MEDITATION:

Duration .... Type...

Time of Day .... Satisfaction Level: 1 2 3 4 5 6 7 8 9 10

Notes: ....

....

Appreciation: (List 5 things you appreciate about your life)

1. ....

2. ....

3. ....

4. ....

5. ....

Gratitude: (List 5 things you are grateful for, which can include future manifestations)

1. ....

2. ....

3. ....

4. ....

5. ....

Set your general intentions for the day:

....

....

....

....

Write five affirmations:

1. ....

2. ....

3. ....

4. ....

5. ....

How did you feel today (or yesterday if you're writing this in the morning)?

....

....

How do you feel now? ....

How do you intend to feel today (or tomorrow if you're writing this in the evening)?

....

....

INSPIRATION:

Did you receive inspiration today (or yesterday if you're writing this in the morning)?

....

....

Describe what you were inspired to do or say ....

....

FOOD EXPERIMENT:

What single item of food did you experiment with today (or yesterday if you're writing this in the morning)? ....

Describe how you felt? ....

....

Does your unique body process this food easily? ....

How did you feel today (or yesterday if you're writing this in the morning)?

....

QUOTE OF THE DAY:

" Your purpose in this life is to expand through experience and fulfill your desires in a joyous manner. You are here to explore. You are here to create desires. You are here to expand with every interest and every experience. You are here to bring forth new thoughts and new ideas. You are here to be a unique expression of source. You come to experience reality in a way that has never been experienced before. In doing so, you wanted guidance in the form of negative and positive emotion." *Joshua*

MEDITATION:

Duration .... Type...

Time of Day .... Satisfaction Level: 1 2 3 4 5 6 7 8 9 10

Notes: ....

....

Appreciation: (List 5 things you appreciate about your life)

1. ....

2. ....

3. ....

4. ....

5. ....

Gratitude: (List 5 things you are grateful for, which can include future manifestations)

1. ....

2. ....

3. ....

4. ....

5. ....

Set your general intentions for the day:

....

....

....

Write five affirmations:

1. ....
2. ....
3. ....
4. ....
5. ....

How did you feel today (or yesterday if you're writing this in the morning)?

....

....

How do you feel now? ....

How do you intend to feel today (or tomorrow if you're writing this in the evening)?

....

....

INSPIRATION:

Did you receive inspiration today (or yesterday if you're writing this in the morning)?

....

....

Describe what you were inspired to do or say ....

....

FOOD EXPERIMENT:

What single item of food did you experiment with today (or yesterday if you're writing this in the morning)? ....

Describe how you felt? ....

....

Does your unique body process this food easily? ....

How did you feel today (or yesterday if you're writing this in the morning)?

....

QUOTE OF THE DAY:

❝ If the fear is irrational, there's nothing real to fear. The fear is false. It might feel real, but like a movie, it's just an illusion. When it comes to irrational fear, the only thing you fear is the negative emotion that comes as a result of trying something new or something out of your comfort zone. As soon as you learn to deal with the fear, by shaping your own positive perception or by analyzing the fear itself, you no longer allow yourself to be limited." *Joshua*

MEDITATION:

Duration .... Type...

Time of Day .... Satisfaction Level: 1 2 3 4 5 6 7 8 9 10

Notes: ....

....

Appreciation: (List 5 things you appreciate about your life)

1. ....

2. ....

3. ....

4. ....

5. ....

Gratitude: (List 5 things you are grateful for, which can include future manifestations)

1. ....

2. ....

3. ....

4. ....

5. ....

Set your general intentions for the day:

....

....

....

Write five affirmations:

1. ....

2. ....

3. ....

4. ....

5. ....

How did you feel today (or yesterday if you're writing this in the morning)?

....

....

How do you feel now? ....

How do you intend to feel today (or tomorrow if you're writing this in the evening)?

....

....

INSPIRATION:

Did you receive inspiration today (or yesterday if you're writing this in the morning)?

....

....

Describe what you were inspired to do or say ....

....

FOOD EXPERIMENT:

What single item of food did you experiment with today (or yesterday if you're writing this in the morning)? ....

Describe how you felt? ....

....

Does your unique body process this food easily? ....

How did you feel today (or yesterday if you're writing this in the morning)?

....

QUOTE OF THE DAY:

❝ Positive emotion is a gift. It lets you know when you're on the right track. Along with the good feeling can come the knowledge that you are moving along just as you had intended and if you can keep this up, you'll receive all that you want." *Joshua*

MEDITATION:

Duration .... Type..

Time of Day .... Satisfaction Level: 1 2 3 4 5 6 7 8 9 10

Notes: ....

....

....

Appreciation: (List 5 things you appreciate about your life)

1. ....

2. ....

3. ....

4. ....

5. ....

Gratitude: (List 5 things you are grateful for, which can include future manifestations)

1. ....

2. ....

3. ....

4. ....

5. ....

Set your general intentions for the day:

....

....

....

....

Write five affirmations:

1. ....

2. ....

3. ....

4. ....

5. ....

How did you feel today (or yesterday if you're writing this in the morning)?

....

....

How do you feel now? ....

How do you intend to feel today (or tomorrow if you're writing this in the evening)?

....

....

INSPIRATION:

Did you receive inspiration today (or yesterday if you're writing this in the morning)?

....

....

Describe what you were inspired to do or say ....

....

FOOD EXPERIMENT:

What single item of food did you experiment with today (or yesterday if you're writing this in the morning)? ....

Describe how you felt? ....

....

Does your unique body process this food easily? ....

How did you feel today (or yesterday if you're writing this in the morning)?

....

QUOTE OF THE DAY:

" If you have come to understand the basic fundamentals of the Law of Attraction, you already realize that you must take into account the vibrational impact of your thoughts, beliefs, words, and actions. When you express out loud that something is wrong, bad, or dangerous, you are simply adding that vibration to your own. Why would you want to bring in something that affects your vibration in a way that causes you to attract that which is not wanted? You would not, but you do it anyway. You think it doesn't matter, but it does." *Joshua*

MEDITATION:

Duration .... Type...

Time of Day .... Satisfaction Level: 1 2 3 4 5 6 7 8 9 10

Notes: ....

....

Appreciation: (List 5 things you appreciate about your life)

1. ....

2. ....

3. ....

4. ....

5. ....

Gratitude: (List 5 things you are grateful for, which can include future manifestations)

1. ....

2. ....

3. ....

4. ....

5. ....

Set your general intentions for the day:

....

....

....

Write five affirmations:

1. ....

2. ....

3. ....

4. ....

5. ....

How did you feel today (or yesterday if you're writing this in the morning)?

....

....

How do you feel now? ....

How do you intend to feel today (or tomorrow if you're writing this in the evening)?

....

....

INSPIRATION:

Did you receive inspiration today (or yesterday if you're writing this in the morning)?

....

....

Describe what you were inspired to do or say ....

....

FOOD EXPERIMENT:

What single item of food did you experiment with today (or yesterday if you're writing this in the morning)? ....

Describe how you felt? ....

....

Does your unique body process this food easily? ....

How did you feel today (or yesterday if you're writing this in the morning)?

....

QUOTE OF THE DAY:

" The first step in an approach to life that works within the laws of the universe is to start talking about things that are wanted. Start talking about things of great interest. Start thinking about new and positive ideas. Start asking to be guided toward conversations, thoughts, and ideas that are pleasing to you. Start intending to find people and conversations that revolve around the things you like." *Joshua*

MEDITATION:

Duration .... Type..

Time of Day .... Satisfaction Level: 1   2   3   4   5   6   7   8   9   10

Notes: ....

....

Appreciation: (List 5 things you appreciate about your life)

1. ....

2. ....

3. ....

4. ....

5. ....

Gratitude: (List 5 things you are grateful for, which can include future manifestations)

1. ....

2. ....

3. ....

4. ....

5. ....

Set your general intentions for the day:

....

....

....

....

Write five affirmations:

1. ....

2. ....

3. ....

4. ....

5. ....

How did you feel today (or yesterday if you're writing this in the morning)?

....

....

How do you feel now? ....

How do you intend to feel today (or tomorrow if you're writing this in the evening)?

....

....

INSPIRATION:

Did you receive inspiration today (or yesterday if you're writing this in the morning)?

....

....

Describe what you were inspired to do or say ....

....

FOOD EXPERIMENT:

What single item of food did you experiment with today (or yesterday if you're writing this in the morning)? ....

Describe how you felt? ....

....

Does your unique body process this food easily? ....

How did you feel today (or yesterday if you're writing this in the morning)?

....

QUOTE OF THE DAY:

" The most common limiting habit is that of complaining. Complaining is powerful focus on that which you think is wrong. You believe that something that has already happened should be different than it is. If you think the conditions in the moment are less than perfect and you wish they would be different, you are reacting from an old paradigm that does not help you in any way." *Joshua*

MEDITATION:

Duration .... Type...

Time of Day .... Satisfaction Level: 1 2 3 4 5 6 7 8 9 10

Notes: ....

....

Appreciation: (List 5 things you appreciate about your life)

1. ....

2. ....

3. ....

4. ....

5. ....

Gratitude: (List 5 things you are grateful for, which can include future manifestations)

1. ....

2. ....

3. ....

4. ....

5. ....

Set your general intentions for the day:

....

....

....

....

Write five affirmations:

1. ....

2. ....

3. ....

4. ....

5. ....

How did you feel today (or yesterday if you're writing this in the morning)?

....

....

How do you feel now? ....

How do you intend to feel today (or tomorrow if you're writing this in the evening)?

....

....

INSPIRATION:

Did you receive inspiration today (or yesterday if you're writing this in the morning)?

....

....

Describe what you were inspired to do or say ....

....

FOOD EXPERIMENT:

What single item of food did you experiment with today (or yesterday if you're writing this in the morning)? ....

Describe how you felt? ....

....

Does your unique body process this food easily? ....

How did you feel today (or yesterday if you're writing this in the morning)?

....

QUOTE OF THE DAY:

" This is an absolute fundamental element of the universe. You cannot escape it. If you think something is wrong or bad, you attract the negative aspects of it and add it to your vibration. If you decide to complain about something, your spoken words are powerful and you create an environment where the subject of your complaint becomes more pronounced and impactful. If you decide to take action against something you think is wrong, you create a monster out of it." *Joshua*

MEDITATION:

Duration .... Type...

Time of Day .... Satisfaction Level: 1 2 3 4 5 6 7 8 9 10

Notes: ....

....

Appreciation: (List 5 things you appreciate about your life)

1. ....

2. ....

3. ....

4. ....

5. ....

Gratitude: (List 5 things you are grateful for, which can include future manifestations)

1. ....

2. ....

3. ....

4. ....

5. ....

Set your general intentions for the day:

....

....

....

Write five affirmations:

1. ....

2. ....

3. ....

4. ....

5. ....

How did you feel today (or yesterday if you're writing this in the morning)?

....

....

How do you feel now? ....

How do you intend to feel today (or tomorrow if you're writing this in the evening)?

....

....

INSPIRATION:

Did you receive inspiration today (or yesterday if you're writing this in the morning)?

....

....

Describe what you were inspired to do or say ....

....

FOOD EXPERIMENT:

What single item of food did you experiment with today (or yesterday if you're writing this in the morning)? ....

Describe how you felt? ....

....

Does your unique body process this food easily? ....

How did you feel today (or yesterday if you're writing this in the morning)?

....

QUOTE OF THE DAY:

" Universal forces are quite powerful. These same forces created worlds, stars, and galaxies. If these forces can create galactic wonders, imagine the power they can wield in your life. When you learn to use universal forces to your benefit, things happen easily. When you live in opposition to these laws, everything is harder. Your approach to life determines whether these forces work for you or against you. Again, it is all up to you." *Joshua*

MEDITATION:

Duration .... Type..

Time of Day .... Satisfaction Level: 1   2   3   4   5   6   7   8   9   10

Notes: ....

....

Appreciation: (List 5 things you appreciate about your life)

1. ....

2. ....

3. ....

4. ....

5. ....

Gratitude: (List 5 things you are grateful for, which can include future manifestations)

1. ....

2. ....

3. ....

4. ....

5. ....

Set your general intentions for the day:

....

....

....

....

Write five affirmations:

1. ....

2. ....

3. ....

4. ....

5. ....

How did you feel today (or yesterday if you're writing this in the morning)?

....

....

How do you feel now? ....

How do you intend to feel today (or tomorrow if you're writing this in the evening)?

....

....

INSPIRATION:

Did you receive inspiration today (or yesterday if you're writing this in the morning)?

....

....

Describe what you were inspired to do or say ....

....

FOOD EXPERIMENT:

What single item of food did you experiment with today (or yesterday if you're writing this in the morning)? ....

Describe how you felt? ....

....

Does your unique body process this food easily? ....

How did you feel today (or yesterday if you're writing this in the morning)?

....

QUOTE OF THE DAY:

❝ Imagine a life where you are completely cared for, loved, and supported from cradle to grave. Everything is provided for you. You can be, do, and have anything you want simply by asking for it. You can explore any aspect of physical reality you choose. Imagine having the ability to bring anything into your life simply by altering your vibration. This is the reality that exists for you now. This is the reality that has always existed for you. This is the design and purpose of this reality. This is the reason you chose to come here." *Joshua*

MEDITATION:

Duration .... Type..

Time of Day .... Satisfaction Level: 1 2 3 4 5 6 7 8 9 10

Notes: ....

....

Appreciation: (List 5 things you appreciate about your life)

1. ....

2. ....

3. ....

4. ....

5. ....

Gratitude: (List 5 things you are grateful for, which can include future manifestations)

1. ....

2. ....

3. ....

4. ....

5. ....

Set your general intentions for the day:

....

....

....

Write five affirmations:

1. ....

2. ....

3. ....

4. ....

5. ....

How did you feel today (or yesterday if you're writing this in the morning)?

....

....

How do you feel now? ....

How do you intend to feel today (or tomorrow if you're writing this in the evening)?

....

....

INSPIRATION:

Did you receive inspiration today (or yesterday if you're writing this in the morning)?

....

....

Describe what you were inspired to do or say ....

....

FOOD EXPERIMENT:

What single item of food did you experiment with today (or yesterday if you're writing this in the morning)? ....

Describe how you felt? ....

....

Does your unique body process this food easily? ....

How did you feel today (or yesterday if you're writing this in the morning)?

....

QUOTE OF THE DAY:

" There is a flow to life and when you relinquish your control, magical things will start happening for you. You do not have to fight this flow; you can simply allow yourself to move in unison with it. The universe knows what you truly want and how to get it. It sends you signals when it's time to act. These signals feel like ideas, thoughts, inspiration, and intuition. It feels right. It feels fun. You want to do it. It seems logical. When you act from inspiration, you are leveraging the forces of the universe and you become highly effective at manifesting that which you desire." *Joshua*

MEDITATION:

Duration .... Type..

Time of Day .... Satisfaction Level: 1 2 3 4 5 6 7 8 9 10

Notes: ....

....

Appreciation: (List 5 things you appreciate about your life)

1. ....

2. ....

3. ....

4. ....

5. ....

Gratitude: (List 5 things you are grateful for, which can include future manifestations)

1. ....

2. ....

3. ....

4. ....

5. ....

Set your general intentions for the day:

....

....

....

Write five affirmations:

1. ....

2. ....

3. ....

4. ....

5. ....

How did you feel today (or yesterday if you're writing this in the morning)?

....

....

How do you feel now? ....

How do you intend to feel today (or tomorrow if you're writing this in the evening)?

....

....

INSPIRATION:

Did you receive inspiration today (or yesterday if you're writing this in the morning)?

....

....

Describe what you were inspired to do or say ....

....

FOOD EXPERIMENT:

What single item of food did you experiment with today (or yesterday if you're writing this in the morning)? ....

Describe how you felt? ....

....

Does your unique body process this food easily? ....

How did you feel today (or yesterday if you're writing this in the morning)?

....

QUOTE OF THE DAY:

" There are many paths that will lead you to the manifestation of your desire and they are all downhill. Nothing you want is uphill. You might work hard to prove you've sacrificed something in order to reach your goal. Your society favors hard work and sacrifice. In your society, these things are respected. You might believe that people simply do not respect those who receive things easily. Yet the ones who go with the flow of life and engage the forces of the universe are the ones who are playing the game effectively. They are doing the real work. The work is an inside job. The universe responds to this work by reflecting it on the outside world." *Joshua*

MEDITATION:

Duration .... Type...

Time of Day .... Satisfaction Level: 1 2 3 4 5 6 7 8 9 10

Notes: ....

....

Appreciation: (List 5 things you appreciate about your life)

1. ....

2. ....

3. ....

4. ....

5. ....

Gratitude: (List 5 things you are grateful for, which can include future manifestations)

1. ....

2. ....

3. ....

4. ....

5. ....

Set your general intentions for the day:

....

....

....

Write five affirmations:

1. ....
2. ....
3. ....
4. ....
5. ....

How did you feel today (or yesterday if you're writing this in the morning)?

....

....

How do you feel now? ....

How do you intend to feel today (or tomorrow if you're writing this in the evening)?

....

....

INSPIRATION:

Did you receive inspiration today (or yesterday if you're writing this in the morning)?

....

....

Describe what you were inspired to do or say ....

....

FOOD EXPERIMENT:

What single item of food did you experiment with today (or yesterday if you're writing this in the morning)? ....

Describe how you felt? ....

....

Does your unique body process this food easily? ....

How did you feel today (or yesterday if you're writing this in the morning)?

....

QUOTE OF THE DAY:

"" When you change who you are, your outer world changes to match the inner you. The outer world, including your body, is a reflection of your inner world. When you seek to change your outer world, you might cause it to change a little, but if you have not changed your inner world, your outer world will gradually change back to reflect how you really feel on the inside. Isn't this good news?" *Joshua*

MEDITATION:

Duration .... Type..

Time of Day .... Satisfaction Level: 1 2 3 4 5 6 7 8 9 10

Notes: ....

....

....

Appreciation: (List 5 things you appreciate about your life)

1. ....

2. ....

3. ....

4. ....

5. ....

Gratitude: (List 5 things you are grateful for, which can include future manifestations)

1. ....

2. ....

3. ....

4. ....

5. ....

Set your general intentions for the day:

....

....

....

Write five affirmations:

1. ....

2. ....

3. ....

4. ....

5. ....

How did you feel today (or yesterday if you're writing this in the morning)?

....

....

How do you feel now? ....

How do you intend to feel today (or tomorrow if you're writing this in the evening)?

....

....

INSPIRATION:

Did you receive inspiration today (or yesterday if you're writing this in the morning)?

....

....

Describe what you were inspired to do or say ....

....

FOOD EXPERIMENT:

What single item of food did you experiment with today (or yesterday if you're writing this in the morning)? ....

Describe how you felt? ....

....

Does your unique body process this food easily? ....

How did you feel today (or yesterday if you're writing this in the morning)?

....

QUOTE OF THE DAY:

" It's not the conditions on the outside that matter; it's always how you feel on the inside that is important. The conditions may change and to the outside observer, they may appear to be improved, but unless the person changes who they are on the inside, the conditions will still represent the same old feelings. The outside may look different, but it will always bring up the same feelings that are being felt on the inside." *Joshua*

MEDITATION:

Duration .... Type...

Time of Day .... Satisfaction Level: 1 2 3 4 5 6 7 8 9 10

Notes: ....

....

Appreciation: (List 5 things you appreciate about your life)

1. ....

2. ....

3. ....

4. ....

5. ....

Gratitude: (List 5 things you are grateful for, which can include future manifestations)

1. ....

2. ....

3. ....

4. ....

5. ....

Set your general intentions for the day:

....

....

....

....

Write five affirmations:

1. ....

2. ....

3. ....

4. ....

5. ....

How did you feel today (or yesterday if you're writing this in the morning)?

....

....

How do you feel now? ....

How do you intend to feel today (or tomorrow if you're writing this in the evening)?

....

....

INSPIRATION:

Did you receive inspiration today (or yesterday if you're writing this in the morning)?

....

....

Describe what you were inspired to do or say ....

....

FOOD EXPERIMENT:

What single item of food did you experiment with today (or yesterday if you're writing this in the morning)? ....

Describe how you felt? ....

....

Does your unique body process this food easily? ....

How did you feel today (or yesterday if you're writing this in the morning)?

....

QUOTE OF THE DAY:

" You are not being asked to change who you are; we are asking you to become who you really are. You are a being of pure positive love and acceptance. Who you really are is one who loves those in your life unconditionally and who accepts the conditions as they are. That's who you really are. If you are behaving in a way that is less than this, you are simply pretending to be someone you are not." *Joshua*

MEDITATION:

Duration .... Type...

Time of Day .... Satisfaction Level: 1 2 3 4 5 6 7 8 9 10

Notes: ....

....

....

Appreciation: (List 5 things you appreciate about your life)

1. ....

2. ....

3. ....

4. ....

5. ....

Gratitude: (List 5 things you are grateful for, which can include future manifestations)

1. ....

2. ....

3. ....

4. ....

5. ....

Set your general intentions for the day:

....

....

....

Write five affirmations:

1. ....

2. ....

3. ....

4. ....

5. ....

How did you feel today (or yesterday if you're writing this in the morning)?

....

....

How do you feel now? ....

How do you intend to feel today (or tomorrow if you're writing this in the evening)?

....

....

INSPIRATION:

Did you receive inspiration today (or yesterday if you're writing this in the morning)?

....

....

Describe what you were inspired to do or say ....

....

FOOD EXPERIMENT:

What single item of food did you experiment with today (or yesterday if you're writing this in the morning)? ....

Describe how you felt? ....

....

Does your unique body process this food easily? ....

How did you feel today (or yesterday if you're writing this in the morning)?

....

QUOTE OF THE DAY:

" You were born into this world with the intention of living a life of joy, freedom, ease, abundance, expansion, and exploration. If your life is not like this now, you are acting in a way that is out of alignment with how you intended to live. It is really quite a lot more difficult to be who you are not than who you really are. It is difficult to pretend to be someone else." *Joshua*

MEDITATION:

Duration .... Type...

Time of Day .... Satisfaction Level: 1 2 3 4 5 6 7 8 9 10

Notes: ....

....

Appreciation: (List 5 things you appreciate about your life)

1. ....

2. ....

3. ....

4. ....

5. ....

Gratitude: (List 5 things you are grateful for, which can include future manifestations)

1. ....

2. ....

3. ....

4. ....

5. ....

Set your general intentions for the day:

....

....

....

....

Write five affirmations:

1. ....

2. ....

3. ....

4. ....

5. ....

How did you feel today (or yesterday if you're writing this in the morning)?

....

....

How do you feel now? ....

How do you intend to feel today (or tomorrow if you're writing this in the evening)?

....

....

INSPIRATION:

Did you receive inspiration today (or yesterday if you're writing this in the morning)?

....

....

Describe what you were inspired to do or say ....

....

FOOD EXPERIMENT:

What single item of food did you experiment with today (or yesterday if you're writing this in the morning)? ....

Describe how you felt? ....

....

Does your unique body process this food easily?..

How did you feel today (or yesterday if you're writing this in the morning)?

....

QUOTE OF THE DAY:

" You came to this world wanting to explore certain aspects of reality and so you chose your parents, the time and place of your birth, and your specific body with all its unique features and attributes. You knew that the environment of your youth would launch you on a trajectory toward where you wanted to go and what you wanted to explore. You chose it all. You chose your unique gifts and talents. You like who you really are, but you may fear showing this to others." *Joshua*

MEDITATION:

Duration .... Type...

Time of Day .... Satisfaction Level: 1 2 3 4 5 6 7 8 9 10

Notes: ....

....

Appreciation: (List 5 things you appreciate about your life)

1. ....

2. ....

3. ....

4. ....

5. ....

Gratitude: (List 5 things you are grateful for, which can include future manifestations)

1. ....

2. ....

3. ....

4. ....

5. ....

Set your general intentions for the day:

....

....

....

Write five affirmations:

1. ....

2. ....

3. ....

4. ....

5. ....

How did you feel today (or yesterday if you're writing this in the morning)?

....

....

How do you feel now? ....

How do you intend to feel today (or tomorrow if you're writing this in the evening)?

....

....

INSPIRATION:

Did you receive inspiration today (or yesterday if you're writing this in the morning)?

....

....

Describe what you were inspired to do or say ....

....

FOOD EXPERIMENT:

What single item of food did you experiment with today (or yesterday if you're writing this in the morning)? ....

Describe how you felt? ....

....

Does your unique body process this food easily? ....

How did you feel today (or yesterday if you're writing this in the morning)?

....

QUOTE OF THE DAY:

" When you change who you are being now to become who you really are, you will find success in all areas of your life. When you are being who you really are, you fully engage the powers of the universe and you are aligned with everything you want. When you suppress who you are out of fear, you disengage some or all of the powers of the universe and you can't really accomplish anything of substance." *Joshua*

MEDITATION:

Duration .... Type...

Time of Day .... Satisfaction Level: 1 2 3 4 5 6 7 8 9 10

Notes: ....

....

....

Appreciation: (List 5 things you appreciate about your life)

1. ....

2. ....

3. ....

4. ....

5. ....

Gratitude: (List 5 things you are grateful for, which can include future manifestations)

1. ....

2. ....

3. ....

4. ....

5. ....

Set your general intentions for the day:

....

....

....

Write five affirmations:

1. ....

2. ....

3. ....

4. ....

5. ....

How did you feel today (or yesterday if you're writing this in the morning)?

....

....

How do you feel now? ....

How do you intend to feel today (or tomorrow if you're writing this in the evening)?

....

....

INSPIRATION:

Did you receive inspiration today (or yesterday if you're writing this in the morning)?

....

....

Describe what you were inspired to do or say ....

....

FOOD EXPERIMENT:

What single item of food did you experiment with today (or yesterday if you're writing this in the morning)? ....

Describe how you felt? ....

....

Does your unique body process this food easily? ....

How did you feel today (or yesterday if you're writing this in the morning)?

....

QUOTE OF THE DAY:

" Your life is created by how you feel on the inside. Your limiting beliefs are a true representation of your fears. These fears are irrational and are therefore false. However, unless you analyze them and prove they are false, they remain true for you. Your life will remain limited. You will not be able to manifest what you desire because your limiting beliefs cause resistance. Realize that negative emotion is simply a gift from the universe that will help you identify limiting beliefs as they arise. The rest is up to you. This is how you make real change. Your reality changes to reflect the real change you've made by doing the work necessary to reduce the intensity of limiting beliefs." *Joshua*

MEDITATION:

Duration .... Type...

Time of Day .... Satisfaction Level: 1 2 3 4 5 6 7 8 9 10

Notes: ....

....

Appreciation: (List 5 things you appreciate about your life)

1. ....

2. ....

3. ....

4. ....

5. ....

Gratitude: (List 5 things you are grateful for, which can include future manifestations)

1. ....

2. ....

3. ....

4. ....

5. ....

Set your general intentions for the day:

....

....

....

Write five affirmations:

1. ....

2. ....

3. ....

4. ....

5. ....

How did you feel today (or yesterday if you're writing this in the morning)?

....

....

How do you feel now? ....

How do you intend to feel today (or tomorrow if you're writing this in the evening)?

....

....

INSPIRATION:

Did you receive inspiration today (or yesterday if you're writing this in the morning)?

....

....

Describe what you were inspired to do or say ....

....

FOOD EXPERIMENT:

What single item of food did you experiment with today (or yesterday if you're writing this in the morning)? ....

Describe how you felt? ....

....

Does your unique body process this food easily? ....

How did you feel today (or yesterday if you're writing this in the morning)?

....

QUOTE OF THE DAY:

" The first inner change you must make is your approach to negative emotion. If you can see negative emotion as a signal flare alerting you to the presence of a limiting belief, you can literally accomplish anything you want. When you shy away from negative emotion because you can't handle the pain and distress, you play it too safe. By playing it safe out of fear of negative emotion, you actually diminish the intensity and strength of your desires." *Joshua*

MEDITATION:

Duration .... Type...

Time of Day .... Satisfaction Level: 1 2 3 4 5 6 7 8 9 10

Notes: ....

....

Appreciation: (List 5 things you appreciate about your life)

1. ....

2. ....

3. ....

4. ....

5. ....

Gratitude: (List 5 things you are grateful for, which can include future manifestations)

1. ....

2. ....

3. ....

4. ....

5. ....

Set your general intentions for the day:

....

....

....

....

Write five affirmations:

1. ....

2. ....

3. ....

4. ....

5. ....

How did you feel today (or yesterday if you're writing this in the morning)?

....

....

How do you feel now? ....

How do you intend to feel today (or tomorrow if you're writing this in the evening)?

....

....

INSPIRATION:

Did you receive inspiration today (or yesterday if you're writing this in the morning)?

....

....

Describe what you were inspired to do or say ....

....

FOOD EXPERIMENT:

What single item of food did you experiment with today (or yesterday if you're writing this in the morning)? ....

Describe how you felt? ....

....

Does your unique body process this food easily? ....

How did you feel today (or yesterday if you're writing this in the morning)?

....

QUOTE OF THE DAY:

" How you react to something sets forth a new path toward a new future. Reaction is a choice. This choice will determine which path you take. When you react negatively, depending on the power of your thoughts, words, and actions, you will go down a path toward what you do not want. When you react negatively, you begin to create negatively. Change your reaction to how you perceive things and you will regain control of your most important creation: your life." *Joshua*

MEDITATION:

Duration .... Type ....

Time of Day .... Satisfaction Level: 1 2 3 4 5 6 7 8 9 10

Notes: ....

....

Appreciation: (List 5 things you appreciate about your life)

1. ....

2. ....

3. ....

4. ....

5. ....

Gratitude: (List 5 things you are grateful for, which can include future manifestations)

1. ....

2. ....

3. ....

4. ....

5. ....

Set your general intentions for the day:

....

....

....

Write five affirmations:

1. ....

2. ....

3. ....

4. ....

5. ....

How did you feel today (or yesterday if you're writing this in the morning)?

....

....

How do you feel now? ....

How do you intend to feel today (or tomorrow if you're writing this in the evening)?

....

....

INSPIRATION:

Did you receive inspiration today (or yesterday if you're writing this in the morning)?

....

....

Describe what you were inspired to do or say ....

....

FOOD EXPERIMENT:

What single item of food did you experiment with today (or yesterday if you're writing this in the morning)? ....

Describe how you felt? ....

....

Does your unique body process this food easily? ....

How did you feel today (or yesterday if you're writing this in the morning)?

....

QUOTE OF THE DAY:

" A reaction is a very powerful statement. It is a declaration. This is good and that is bad. How you react to something causes a shift in your consciousness. Your reaction creates the reception of certain specific channels of thought. It's like tuning into a radio station. There are many, many channels to choose from. Negative reactions give you access to many varieties of fear-based channels. Positive reactions give you access to the love-based channels." *Joshua*

MEDITATION:

Duration .... Type...

Time of Day .... Satisfaction Level: 1 2 3 4 5 6 7 8 9 10

Notes: ....

....

Appreciation: (List 5 things you appreciate about your life)

1. ....

2. ....

3. ....

4. ....

5. ....

Gratitude: (List 5 things you are grateful for, which can include future manifestations)

1. ....

2. ....

3. ....

4. ....

5. ....

Set your general intentions for the day:

....

....

....

Write five affirmations:

1. ....

2. ....

3. ....

4. ....

5. ....

How did you feel today (or yesterday if you're writing this in the morning)?

....

....

How do you feel now? ....

How do you intend to feel today (or tomorrow if you're writing this in the evening)?

....

....

INSPIRATION:

Did you receive inspiration today (or yesterday if you're writing this in the morning)?

....

....

Describe what you were inspired to do or say ....

....

FOOD EXPERIMENT:

What single item of food did you experiment with today (or yesterday if you're writing this in the morning)? ....

Describe how you felt? ....

....

Does your unique body process this food easily? ....

How did you feel today (or yesterday if you're writing this in the morning)?

....

QUOTE OF THE DAY:

" It all starts by changing the way you react to everything outside of you. Don't try to change the outer conditions; go inside and change your own channel. Stop and analyze your thoughts. Are they leading you to action that aligns with love or fear? If the actions are based in fear, you will create what you do not want. If the actions are based in love, you are consciously creating the life you prefer." *Joshua*

MEDITATION:

Duration .... Type..

Time of Day .... Satisfaction Level: 1 2 3 4 5 6 7 8 9 10

Notes: ....

....

....

Appreciation: (List 5 things you appreciate about your life)

1. ....

2. ....

3. ....

4. ....

5. ....

Gratitude: (List 5 things you are grateful for, which can include future manifestations)

1. ....

2. ....

3. ....

4. ....

5. ....

Set your general intentions for the day:

....

....

....

Write five affirmations:

1. ....

2. ....

3. ....

4. ....

5. ....

How did you feel today (or yesterday if you're writing this in the morning)?

....

....

How do you feel now? ....

How do you intend to feel today (or tomorrow if you're writing this in the evening)?

....

....

INSPIRATION:

Did you receive inspiration today (or yesterday if you're writing this in the morning)?

....

....

Describe what you were inspired to do or say ....

....

FOOD EXPERIMENT:

What single item of food did you experiment with today (or yesterday if you're writing this in the morning)? ....

Describe how you felt? ....

....

Does your unique body process this food easily? ....

How did you feel today (or yesterday if you're writing this in the morning)?

....

QUOTE OF THE DAY:

66 Every thought you think is a point of creation. Every thought affects what you are creating. Every thought has the power to add to the momentum or to slow it down. You attract thoughts and then you think them. You have total control over the thoughts you think even though you might believe otherwise." *Joshua*

MEDITATION:

Duration .... Type..

Time of Day .... Satisfaction Level: 1   2   3   4   5   6   7   8   9   10

Notes: ....

....

....

Appreciation: (List 5 things you appreciate about your life)

1. ....

2. ....

3. ....

4. ....

5. ....

Gratitude: (List 5 things you are grateful for, which can include future manifestations)

1. ....

2. ....

3. ....

4. ....

5. ....

Set your general intentions for the day:

....

....

....

....

Write five affirmations:

1. ....

2. ....

3. ....

4. ....

5. ....

How did you feel today (or yesterday if you're writing this in the morning)?

....

....

How do you feel now? ....

How do you intend to feel today (or tomorrow if you're writing this in the evening)?

....

....

INSPIRATION:

Did you receive inspiration today (or yesterday if you're writing this in the morning)?

....

....

Describe what you were inspired to do or say ....

....

FOOD EXPERIMENT:

What single item of food did you experiment with today (or yesterday if you're writing this in the morning)? ....

Describe how you felt? ....

....

Does your unique body process this food easily? ....

How did you feel today (or yesterday if you're writing this in the morning)?

....

QUOTE OF THE DAY:

" All the thoughts and ideas that have ever been thought still exist. All the thoughts and ideas that ever will be thought also exist. Thoughts that have not yet been thought are at frequencies that have not yet been reached. They may be reached tomorrow or never, but they still exist. When you get an original idea, it's not that you created the idea, it's just that you were the first to reach the vibrational frequency of the idea." *Joshua*

MEDITATION:

Duration .... Type..

Time of Day .... Satisfaction Level: 1 2 3 4 5 6 7 8 9 10

Notes: ....

....

Appreciation: (List 5 things you appreciate about your life)

1. ....

2. ....

3. ....

4. ....

5. ....

Gratitude: (List 5 things you are grateful for, which can include future manifestations)

1. ....

2. ....

3. ....

4. ....

5. ....

Set your general intentions for the day:

....

....

....

....

Write five affirmations:

1. ....

2. ....

3. ....

4. ....

5. ....

How did you feel today (or yesterday if you're writing this in the morning)?

....

....

How do you feel now? ....

How do you intend to feel today (or tomorrow if you're writing this in the evening)?

....

....

INSPIRATION:

Did you receive inspiration today (or yesterday if you're writing this in the morning)?

....

....

Describe what you were inspired to do or say ....

....

FOOD EXPERIMENT:

What single item of food did you experiment with today (or yesterday if you're writing this in the morning)? ....

Describe how you felt? ....

....

Does your unique body process this food easily? ....

How did you feel today (or yesterday if you're writing this in the morning)?

....

DAY 45: _____ / _____ / _____   M   T   W   T   F   S   S

QUOTE OF THE DAY:

" If you could control the quality of every single thought that comes to you, what would that really mean? It would mean that you were a deliberate creator of your life. Since your thoughts create your reality, if you could maintain a vibration where you received only high-vibrational thoughts, your life would be created in a way that perfectly aligned with the quality of thoughts you were thinking. You would enjoy a high-quality life experience." *Joshua*

MEDITATION:

Duration .... Type...

Time of Day .... Satisfaction Level: 1 2 3 4 5 6 7 8 9 10

Notes: ....

....

Appreciation: (List 5 things you appreciate about your life)

1. ....

2. ....

3. ....

4. ....

5. ....

Gratitude: (List 5 things you are grateful for, which can include future manifestations)

1. ....

2. ....

3. ....

4. ....

5. ....

Set your general intentions for the day:

....

....

....

Write five affirmations:

1. ....

2. ....

3. ....

4. ....

5. ....

How did you feel today (or yesterday if you're writing this in the morning)?

....

....

How do you feel now? ....

How do you intend to feel today (or tomorrow if you're writing this in the evening)?

....

....

INSPIRATION:

Did you receive inspiration today (or yesterday if you're writing this in the morning)?

....

....

Describe what you were inspired to do or say ....

....

FOOD EXPERIMENT:

What single item of food did you experiment with today (or yesterday if you're writing this in the morning)? ....

Describe how you felt? ....

....

Does your unique body process this food easily? ....

How did you feel today (or yesterday if you're writing this in the morning)?

....

DAY 46: _____ / _____ / _____   M T W T F S S

QUOTE OF THE DAY:

66 Whenever you think a low-quality thought, your guidance system kicks in and sends you a signal in the form of negative emotion. You don't have to pay attention to your thoughts because your guidance system is constantly aware of every thought you are thinking and if you choose a thought that does not align with what you want, you will be notified." *Joshua*

MEDITATION:

Duration .... Type...

Time of Day .... Satisfaction Level: 1 2 3 4 5 6 7 8 9 10

Notes: ....

....

Appreciation: (List 5 things you appreciate about your life)

 1. ....

 2. ....

 3. ....

 4. ....

 5. ....

Gratitude: (List 5 things you are grateful for, which can include future manifestations)

 1. ....

 2. ....

 3. ....

 4. ....

 5. ....

Set your general intentions for the day:

....

....

....

....

Write five affirmations:

1. ....

2. ....

3. ....

4. ....

5. ....

How did you feel today (or yesterday if you're writing this in the morning)?

....

....

How do you feel now? ....

How do you intend to feel today (or tomorrow if you're writing this in the evening)?

....

....

INSPIRATION:

Did you receive inspiration today (or yesterday if you're writing this in the morning)?

....

....

Describe what you were inspired to do or say ....

....

FOOD EXPERIMENT:

What single item of food did you experiment with today (or yesterday if you're writing this in the morning)? ....

Describe how you felt? ....

....

Does your unique body process this food easily?..

How did you feel today (or yesterday if you're writing this in the morning)?

....

QUOTE OF THE DAY:

" When you feel irrational fear, the fear is false so you are fabricating a perspective that causes you to feel fear. You could just as easily don a perspective that allows you to feel good. But the fear causes you to adopt the limiting perspective. Since you made it all up anyway, since you cannot know which path the universe is taking you, since you cannot know how it will all unfold, why not substitute fear for faith?" *Joshua*

MEDITATION:

Duration .... Type...

Time of Day .... Satisfaction Level: 1 2 3 4 5 6 7 8 9 10

Notes: ....

....

....

Appreciation: (List 5 things you appreciate about your life)

1. ....

2. ....

3. ....

4. ....

5. ....

Gratitude: (List 5 things you are grateful for, which can include future manifestations)

1. ....

2. ....

3. ....

4. ....

5. ....

Set your general intentions for the day:

....

....

....

Write five affirmations:

1. ....

2. ....

3. ....

4. ....

5. ....

How did you feel today (or yesterday if you're writing this in the morning)?

....

....

How do you feel now? ....

How do you intend to feel today (or tomorrow if you're writing this in the evening)?

....

....

INSPIRATION:

Did you receive inspiration today (or yesterday if you're writing this in the morning)?

....

....

Describe what you were inspired to do or say ....

....

FOOD EXPERIMENT:

What single item of food did you experiment with today (or yesterday if you're writing this in the morning)? ....

Describe how you felt? ....

....

Does your unique body process this food easily? ....

How did you feel today (or yesterday if you're writing this in the morning)?

....

QUOTE OF THE DAY:

❝ The first time you were dumped in a relationship, you felt pain. You might have thought at the time, 'If only the person loved me, things would have been different.' Looking back, would you really have wanted to stay with that person or could you appreciate the growth that that relationship created? You think you know what you want, but you really don't. When you try to create your own life as you see a specific path in your imagination, you are simply resisting the path that the universe has chosen for you." *Joshua*

MEDITATION:

Duration .... Type..

Time of Day .... Satisfaction Level: 1 2 3 4 5 6 7 8 9 10

Notes: ....

....

Appreciation: (List 5 things you appreciate about your life)

1. ....

2. ....

3. ....

4. ....

5. ....

Gratitude: (List 5 things you are grateful for, which can include future manifestations)

1. ....

2. ....

3. ....

4. ....

5. ....

Set your general intentions for the day:

....

....

....

Write five affirmations:

1. ....

2. ....

3. ....

4. ....

5. ....

How did you feel today (or yesterday if you're writing this in the morning)?

....

....

How do you feel now? ....

How do you intend to feel today (or tomorrow if you're writing this in the evening)?

....

....

INSPIRATION:

Did you receive inspiration today (or yesterday if you're writing this in the morning)?

....

....

Describe what you were inspired to do or say ....

....

FOOD EXPERIMENT:

What single item of food did you experiment with today (or yesterday if you're writing this in the morning)? ....

Describe how you felt? ....

....

Does your unique body process this food easily? ....

How did you feel today (or yesterday if you're writing this in the morning)?

....

QUOTE OF THE DAY:

66 You must have a set of personal experiences in order to become the version of you that will be ready for your desire. You must undergo a transformation. All of these experiences are for your higher good. They are all part of the transformation process. Most of the experiences will seem good and some will seem bad, but if you can understand that they are all for your higher good and they are all part of the transformation process, then you can begin to judge them all as good rather than seeing some of them as wrong." *Joshua*

MEDITATION:

Duration .... Type...

Time of Day .... Satisfaction Level: 1 2 3 4 5 6 7 8 9 10

Notes: ....

....

Appreciation: (List 5 things you appreciate about your life)

1. ....

2. ....

3. ....

4. ....

5. ....

Gratitude: (List 5 things you are grateful for, which can include future manifestations)

1. ....

2. ....

3. ....

4. ....

5. ....

Set your general intentions for the day:

....

....

....

Write five affirmations:

1. ....

2. ....

3. ....

4. ....

5. ....

How did you feel today (or yesterday if you're writing this in the morning)?

....

....

How do you feel now? ....

How do you intend to feel today (or tomorrow if you're writing this in the evening)?

....

....

INSPIRATION:

Did you receive inspiration today (or yesterday if you're writing this in the morning)?

....

....

Describe what you were inspired to do or say ....

....

FOOD EXPERIMENT:

What single item of food did you experiment with today (or yesterday if you're writing this in the morning)? ....

Describe how you felt? ....

....

Does your unique body process this food easily? ....

How did you feel today (or yesterday if you're writing this in the morning)?

....

QUOTE OF THE DAY:

" Your fabricated persona is comprised of certain specific personality traits, physical features, and mental constructs. The one thing to always keep in mind is that your persona is not true. Who you think you are is not who you really are. Your persona is a smaller and limited version of who you really are. In actuality, it's minuscule compared to the magnificence that is you. This is true of everyone." *Joshua*

MEDITATION:

Duration .... Type...

Time of Day .... Satisfaction Level: 1 2 3 4 5 6 7 8 9 10

Notes: ....

....

Appreciation: (List 5 things you appreciate about your life)

1. ....

2. ....

3. ....

4. ....

5. ....

Gratitude: (List 5 things you are grateful for, which can include future manifestations)

1. ....

2. ....

3. ....

4. ....

5. ....

Set your general intentions for the day:

....

....

....

....

Write five affirmations:

1. ....

2. ....

3. ....

4. ....

5. ....

How did you feel today (or yesterday if you're writing this in the morning)?

....

....

How do you feel now? ....

How do you intend to feel today (or tomorrow if you're writing this in the evening)?

....

....

INSPIRATION:

Did you receive inspiration today (or yesterday if you're writing this in the morning)?

....

....

Describe what you were inspired to do or say ....

....

FOOD EXPERIMENT:

What single item of food did you experiment with today (or yesterday if you're writing this in the morning)? ....

Describe how you felt? ....

....

Does your unique body process this food easily?..

How did you feel today (or yesterday if you're writing this in the morning)?

....

QUOTE OF THE DAY:

" Intend to feel good. What could be a more powerful intention than that? Everything you think you want is wanted in the hopes that the result will feel good. If you simply intend to feel good, then you will receive experiences that feel good. It doesn't really need to be any more specific than that. The feeling of love, peace, success, security, faith, trust, abundance, freedom, prosperity, relief, ease, and well-being all feel good. If you feel good, then what else is needed?" *Joshua*

MEDITATION:

Duration .... Type...

Time of Day .... Satisfaction Level: 1 2 3 4 5 6 7 8 9 10

Notes: ....

....

Appreciation: (List 5 things you appreciate about your life)

1. ....

2. ....

3. ....

4. ....

5. ....

Gratitude: (List 5 things you are grateful for, which can include future manifestations)

1. ....

2. ....

3. ....

4. ....

5. ....

Set your general intentions for the day:

....

....

....

Write five affirmations:

1. ....
2. ....
3. ....
4. ....
5. ....

How did you feel today (or yesterday if you're writing this in the morning)?

....

....

How do you feel now? ....

How do you intend to feel today (or tomorrow if you're writing this in the evening)?

....

....

INSPIRATION:

Did you receive inspiration today (or yesterday if you're writing this in the morning)?

....

....

Describe what you were inspired to do or say ....

....

FOOD EXPERIMENT:

What single item of food did you experiment with today (or yesterday if you're writing this in the morning)? ....

Describe how you felt? ....

....

Does your unique body process this food easily? ....

How did you feel today (or yesterday if you're writing this in the morning)?

....

QUOTE OF THE DAY:

" When you set your intentions, you align your focus of attention to what is wanted. No one intends to do anything that is not in their best interests; it's just that they do not set the intention in the first place. Setting intentions can become a habit that will help you create the life you truly desire." *Joshua*

MEDITATION:

Duration .... Type...

Time of Day .... Satisfaction Level: 1 2 3 4 5 6 7 8 9 10

Notes: ....

....

....

Appreciation: (List 5 things you appreciate about your life)

1. ....

2. ....

3. ....

4. ....

5. ....

Gratitude: (List 5 things you are grateful for, which can include future manifestations)

1. ....

2. ....

3. ....

4. ....

5. ....

Set your general intentions for the day:

....

....

....

....

Write five affirmations:

1. ....

2. ....

3. ....

4. ....

5. ....

How did you feel today (or yesterday if you're writing this in the morning)?

....

....

How do you feel now? ....

How do you intend to feel today (or tomorrow if you're writing this in the evening)?

....

....

INSPIRATION:

Did you receive inspiration today (or yesterday if you're writing this in the morning)?

....

....

Describe what you were inspired to do or say ....

....

FOOD EXPERIMENT:

What single item of food did you experiment with today (or yesterday if you're writing this in the morning)? ....

Describe how you felt? ....

....

Does your unique body process this food easily? ....

How did you feel today (or yesterday if you're writing this in the morning)?

....

DAY 53: _____ / _____ / _____   M T W T F S S

QUOTE OF THE DAY:

" This is the most important thing we have to say. Make it your primary intention to feel good and then all thoughts, ideas, words, and actions that are attracted to you will be in complete alignment with who you really are and what you really want." *Joshua*

MEDITATION:

Duration .... Type..

Time of Day .... Satisfaction Level: 1 2 3 4 5 6 7 8 9 10

Notes: ....

....

....

Appreciation: (List 5 things you appreciate about your life)

1. ....

2. ....

3. ....

4. ....

5. ....

Gratitude: (List 5 things you are grateful for, which can include future manifestations)

1. ....

2. ....

3. ....

4. ....

5. ....

Set your general intentions for the day:

....

....

....

....

Write five affirmations:

1. ....

2. ....

3. ....

4. ....

5. ....

How did you feel today (or yesterday if you're writing this in the morning)?

....

....

How do you feel now? ....

How do you intend to feel today (or tomorrow if you're writing this in the evening)?

....

....

INSPIRATION:

Did you receive inspiration today (or yesterday if you're writing this in the morning)?

....

....

Describe what you were inspired to do or say ....

....

FOOD EXPERIMENT:

What single item of food did you experiment with today (or yesterday if you're writing this in the morning)? ....

Describe how you felt? ....

....

Does your unique body process this food easily? ....

How did you feel today (or yesterday if you're writing this in the morning)?

....

QUOTE OF THE DAY:

" When you enter the state of allowing, you are receptive. You put yourself in the mode of receiving. You are attracting by the very creation of your desire and in order for your desire to manifest into your reality, you must receive it. Think of anything you want as a gift. You ask for the gift and you allow the gift to be given. You do not physically create the gift. All you do is birth the desire and expect the universe to bring it to you." *Joshua*

MEDITATION:

Duration .... Type...

Time of Day .... Satisfaction Level: 1 2 3 4 5 6 7 8 9 10

Notes: ....

....

Appreciation: (List 5 things you appreciate about your life)

1. ....

2. ....

3. ....

4. ....

5. ....

Gratitude: (List 5 things you are grateful for, which can include future manifestations)

1. ....

2. ....

3. ....

4. ....

5. ....

Set your general intentions for the day:

....

....

....

....

Write five affirmations:

1. ....

2. ....

3. ....

4. ....

5. ....

How did you feel today (or yesterday if you're writing this in the morning)?

....

....

How do you feel now? ....

How do you intend to feel today (or tomorrow if you're writing this in the evening)?

....

....

INSPIRATION:

Did you receive inspiration today (or yesterday if you're writing this in the morning)?

....

....

Describe what you were inspired to do or say ....

....

FOOD EXPERIMENT:

What single item of food did you experiment with today (or yesterday if you're writing this in the morning)? ....

Describe how you felt? ....

....

Does your unique body process this food easily? ....

How did you feel today (or yesterday if you're writing this in the morning)?

....

QUOTE OF THE DAY:

" Allowing is natural. In a natural world, free from the influences of your fearful society, you would live a life of ease, conjuring up one desire after another and expecting those desires to manifest in the most elegant manner imaginable. Your life would be one of ease, acceptance, unconditional love, and complete freedom. You could have, be, and do anything you dreamed of. It would be paradise." *Joshua*

MEDITATION:

Duration .... Type..

Time of Day .... Satisfaction Level: 1   2   3   4   5   6   7   8   9   10

Notes: ....

....

Appreciation: (List 5 things you appreciate about your life)

1. ....

2. ....

3. ....

4. ....

5. ....

Gratitude: (List 5 things you are grateful for, which can include future manifestations)

1. ....

2. ....

3. ....

4. ....

5. ....

Set your general intentions for the day:

....

....

....

....

Write five affirmations:

1. ....

2. ....

3. ....

4. ....

5. ....

How did you feel today (or yesterday if you're writing this in the morning)?

....

....

How do you feel now? ....

How do you intend to feel today (or tomorrow if you're writing this in the evening)?

....

....

INSPIRATION:

Did you receive inspiration today (or yesterday if you're writing this in the morning)?

....

....

Describe what you were inspired to do or say ....

....

FOOD EXPERIMENT:

What single item of food did you experiment with today (or yesterday if you're writing this in the morning)? ....

Describe how you felt? ....

....

Does your unique body process this food easily? ....

How did you feel today (or yesterday if you're writing this in the morning)?

....

QUOTE OF THE DAY:

❝ We want to tell you that there is a better way. There is an approach to life that is not defined by what you are doing, but rather by how you are being. Being is a state based in the present moment. How you are being will create what unfolds in your future. If you are being worried in this moment, you will resonate with those things you are worried about. If you are being trusting, you will resonate with that which you hope for." *Joshua*

MEDITATION:

Duration .... Type...

Time of Day .... Satisfaction Level: 1 2 3 4 5 6 7 8 9 10

Notes: ....

....

....

Appreciation: (List 5 things you appreciate about your life)

1. ....

2. ....

3. ....

4. ....

5. ....

Gratitude: (List 5 things you are grateful for, which can include future manifestations)

1. ....

2. ....

3. ....

4. ....

5. ....

Set your general intentions for the day:

....

....

....

Write five affirmations:

1. ....

2. ....

3. ....

4. ....

5. ....

How did you feel today (or yesterday if you're writing this in the morning)?

....

....

How do you feel now? ....

How do you intend to feel today (or tomorrow if you're writing this in the evening)?

....

....

INSPIRATION:

Did you receive inspiration today (or yesterday if you're writing this in the morning)?

....

....

Describe what you were inspired to do or say ....

....

FOOD EXPERIMENT:

What single item of food did you experiment with today (or yesterday if you're writing this in the morning)? ....

Describe how you felt? ....

....

Does your unique body process this food easily? ....

How did you feel today (or yesterday if you're writing this in the morning)?

....

QUOTE OF THE DAY:

❝ When you view something as wrong, out of place, or inconsistent with what you want, you are resisting it. It is not wrong for you; it only seems wrong. You think you don't want it, but all you are doing is resisting it. If you gave up your resistance, the thing would present its message to you and then leave your reality because it is no longer necessary." *Joshua*

MEDITATION:

Duration .... Type..

Time of Day .... Satisfaction Level: 1 2 3 4 5 6 7 8 9 10

Notes: ....

....

Appreciation: (List 5 things you appreciate about your life)

1. ....

2. ....

3. ....

4. ....

5. ....

Gratitude: (List 5 things you are grateful for, which can include future manifestations)

1. ....

2. ....

3. ....

4. ....

5. ....

Set your general intentions for the day:

....

....

....

....

Write five affirmations:

1. ....

2. ....

3. ....

4. ....

5. ....

How did you feel today (or yesterday if you're writing this in the morning)?

....

....

How do you feel now? ....

How do you intend to feel today (or tomorrow if you're writing this in the evening)?

....

....

INSPIRATION:

Did you receive inspiration today (or yesterday if you're writing this in the morning)?

....

....

Describe what you were inspired to do or say ....

....

FOOD EXPERIMENT:

What single item of food did you experiment with today (or yesterday if you're writing this in the morning)? ....

Describe how you felt? ....

....

Does your unique body process this food easily? ....

How did you feel today (or yesterday if you're writing this in the morning)?

....

QUOTE OF THE DAY:

" No one is going to help you but you. It's up to you to discover how the universe works, how your beliefs work, and how you can alter them through the art of analysis. There is no true support group. Most people you know are committed to the old approach to life. This approach, where you make things happen and you ignore negative emotion, does not work. They will counsel you and persuade you to keep trying what is not working; however, you have found a new approach." *Joshua*

MEDITATION:

Duration ....   Type...

Time of Day ....   Satisfaction Level: 1   2   3   4   5   6   7   8   9   10

Notes: ....

....

Appreciation: (List 5 things you appreciate about your life)

1. ....

2. ....

3. ....

4. ....

5. ....

Gratitude: (List 5 things you are grateful for, which can include future manifestations)

1. ....

2. ....

3. ....

4. ....

5. ....

Set your general intentions for the day:

....

....

....

Write five affirmations:

1. ....
2. ....
3. ....
4. ....
5. ....

How did you feel today (or yesterday if you're writing this in the morning)?

....

....

How do you feel now? ....

How do you intend to feel today (or tomorrow if you're writing this in the evening)?

....

....

INSPIRATION:

Did you receive inspiration today (or yesterday if you're writing this in the morning)?

....

....

Describe what you were inspired to do or say ....

....

FOOD EXPERIMENT:

What single item of food did you experiment with today (or yesterday if you're writing this in the morning)? ....

Describe how you felt? ....

....

Does your unique body process this food easily? ....

How did you feel today (or yesterday if you're writing this in the morning)?

....

QUOTE OF THE DAY:

❝ The new approach to life is one of allowing, not pushing against. It is one of receiving, not taking. It is one of patience, not performance. In this approach to life, you focus your power of attention on what you prefer and how you feel. This is a feeling reality and the only thing that really matters is how you feel. Do you feel good? Then that is what matters. Are you experiencing negative emotion? Then stop and analyze the fear at the basis of the limiting belief and find a new, higher perspective that creates the feeling of relief." *Joshua*

MEDITATION:

Duration .... Type...

Time of Day .... Satisfaction Level: 1 2 3 4 5 6 7 8 9 10

Notes: ....

....

Appreciation: (List 5 things you appreciate about your life)

1. ....

2. ....

3. ....

4. ....

5. ....

Gratitude: (List 5 things you are grateful for, which can include future manifestations)

1. ....

2. ....

3. ....

4. ....

5. ....

Set your general intentions for the day:

....

....

....

Write five affirmations:

1. ....
2. ....
3. ....
4. ....
5. ....

How did you feel today (or yesterday if you're writing this in the morning)?

....

....

How do you feel now? ....

How do you intend to feel today (or tomorrow if you're writing this in the evening)?

....

....

INSPIRATION:

Did you receive inspiration today (or yesterday if you're writing this in the morning)?

....

....

Describe what you were inspired to do or say ....

....

FOOD EXPERIMENT:

What single item of food did you experiment with today (or yesterday if you're writing this in the morning)? ....

Describe how you felt? ....

....

Does your unique body process this food easily? ....

How did you feel today (or yesterday if you're writing this in the morning)?

....

QUOTE OF THE DAY:

" In the new approach to life, your goal is to feel good now, not some time in the future when your dream manifests into your reality. Feel good now and you create an environment where your dreams can manifest. It doesn't matter if you're going to feel good in the future unless you can feel good in the present moment. Don't do anything unless it feels good now. If it isn't fun, interesting, or enjoyable, don't do it. Do things that are appealing or wait for inspiration to strike." *Joshua*

MEDITATION:

Duration .... Type...

Time of Day .... Satisfaction Level: 1 2 3 4 5 6 7 8 9 10

Notes: ....

....

Appreciation: (List 5 things you appreciate about your life)

1. ....

2. ....

3. ....

4. ....

5. ....

Gratitude: (List 5 things you are grateful for, which can include future manifestations)

1. ....

2. ....

3. ....

4. ....

5. ....

Set your general intentions for the day:

....

....

....

Write five affirmations:

1. ....

2. ....

3. ....

4. ....

5. ....

How did you feel today (or yesterday if you're writing this in the morning)?

....

....

How do you feel now? ....

How do you intend to feel today (or tomorrow if you're writing this in the evening)?

....

....

INSPIRATION:

Did you receive inspiration today (or yesterday if you're writing this in the morning)?

....

....

Describe what you were inspired to do or say ....

....

FOOD EXPERIMENT:

What single item of food did you experiment with today (or yesterday if you're writing this in the morning)? ....

Describe how you felt? ....

....

Does your unique body process this food easily? ....

How did you feel today (or yesterday if you're writing this in the morning)?

....

QUOTE OF THE DAY:

" If you are to fail and you judge failure as a bad thing, then your persona runs the risk of being damaged by failure. Your ego will not allow this. Your ego is there to protect the persona. Your ego will keep you from doing anything where you might fail just so it can maintain the status of the persona. Your ego is the reason you don't want to leave your comfort zone." *Joshua*

MEDITATION:

Duration .... Type..

Time of Day .... Satisfaction Level: 1 2 3 4 5 6 7 8 9 10

Notes: ....

....

....

Appreciation: (List 5 things you appreciate about your life)

1. ....

2. ....

3. ....

4. ....

5. ....

Gratitude: (List 5 things you are grateful for, which can include future manifestations)

1. ....

2. ....

3. ....

4. ....

5. ....

Set your general intentions for the day:

....

....

....

Write five affirmations:

1. ....

2. ....

3. ....

4. ....

5. ....

How did you feel today (or yesterday if you're writing this in the morning)?

....

....

How do you feel now? ....

How do you intend to feel today (or tomorrow if you're writing this in the evening)?

....

....

INSPIRATION:

Did you receive inspiration today (or yesterday if you're writing this in the morning)?

....

....

Describe what you were inspired to do or say ....

....

FOOD EXPERIMENT:

What single item of food did you experiment with today (or yesterday if you're writing this in the morning)? ....

Describe how you felt? ....

....

Does your unique body process this food easily? ....

How did you feel today (or yesterday if you're writing this in the morning)?

....

QUOTE OF THE DAY:

" Experiment with your belief system. Allow your beliefs to be challenged. Experiment with your mood. Allow your mood to be elevated. Experiment with your feelings. Think about how you feel and see if you can't make yourself feel better. Experiment with your ability to manifest things. See if you notice when the time is aligned on a digital clock. Take notice that when you elevate your mood you encounter friendly people. Notice that when you set your intentions, everything just falls into place." *Joshua*

MEDITATION:

Duration .... Type..

Time of Day .... Satisfaction Level: 1 2 3 4 5 6 7 8 9 10

Notes: ....

....

Appreciation: (List 5 things you appreciate about your life)

1. ....

2. ....

3. ....

4. ....

5. ....

Gratitude: (List 5 things you are grateful for, which can include future manifestations)

1. ....

2. ....

3. ....

4. ....

5. ....

Set your general intentions for the day:

....

....

....

Write five affirmations:

1. ....
2. ....
3. ....
4. ....
5. ....

How did you feel today (or yesterday if you're writing this in the morning)?

....

....

How do you feel now? ....

How do you intend to feel today (or tomorrow if you're writing this in the evening)?

....

....

INSPIRATION:

Did you receive inspiration today (or yesterday if you're writing this in the morning)?

....

....

Describe what you were inspired to do or say ....

....

FOOD EXPERIMENT:

What single item of food did you experiment with today (or yesterday if you're writing this in the morning)? ....

Describe how you felt? ....

....

Does your unique body process this food easily? ....

How did you feel today (or yesterday if you're writing this in the morning)?

....

QUOTE OF THE DAY:

❝ How you feel is the only thing that really matters, because this is a feeling reality and all you are ever doing is feeling something. No matter where you are, who you're with, or what you are physically doing, all you are doing is feeling. If you can create the intention and desire to feel good, then due to the Law of Attraction, you will attract more good-feeling experiences and things. Your only work is to work on feeling as good as you can as often as you can." *Joshua*

MEDITATION:

Duration .... Type..

Time of Day .... Satisfaction Level: 1 2 3 4 5 6 7 8 9 10

Notes: ....

....

Appreciation: (List 5 things you appreciate about your life)

1. ....

2. ....

3. ....

4. ....

5. ....

Gratitude: (List 5 things you are grateful for, which can include future manifestations)

1. ....

2. ....

3. ....

4. ....

5. ....

Set your general intentions for the day:

....

....

....

Write five affirmations:

1. ....

2. ....

3. ....

4. ....

5. ....

How did you feel today (or yesterday if you're writing this in the morning)?

....

....

How do you feel now? ....

How do you intend to feel today (or tomorrow if you're writing this in the evening)?

....

....

INSPIRATION:

Did you receive inspiration today (or yesterday if you're writing this in the morning)?

....

....

Describe what you were inspired to do or say ....

....

FOOD EXPERIMENT:

What single item of food did you experiment with today (or yesterday if you're writing this in the morning)? ....

Describe how you felt? ....

....

Does your unique body process this food easily? ....

How did you feel today (or yesterday if you're writing this in the morning)?

....

QUOTE OF THE DAY:

" Your senses bring you feedback about the physical world, but they don't cause how you feel. You determine how you feel by your own interpretation of the feedback you are receiving. If you feel good, you are interpreting your reality from a perspective that allows you to feel good. If you feel bad, you are looking at the outside conditions from a limited perspective that causes you to feel bad. It's your perspective, so it's always your choice." *Joshua*

MEDITATION:

Duration .... Type...

Time of Day .... Satisfaction Level: 1 2 3 4 5 6 7 8 9 10

Notes: ....

....

Appreciation: (List 5 things you appreciate about your life)

1. ....

2. ....

3. ....

4. ....

5. ....

Gratitude: (List 5 things you are grateful for, which can include future manifestations)

1. ....

2. ....

3. ....

4. ....

5. ....

Set your general intentions for the day:

....

....

....

....

Write five affirmations:

1. ....

2. ....

3. ....

4. ....

5. ....

How did you feel today (or yesterday if you're writing this in the morning)?

....

....

How do you feel now? ....

How do you intend to feel today (or tomorrow if you're writing this in the evening)?

....

....

INSPIRATION:

Did you receive inspiration today (or yesterday if you're writing this in the morning)?

....

....

Describe what you were inspired to do or say ....

....

FOOD EXPERIMENT:

What single item of food did you experiment with today (or yesterday if you're writing this in the morning)? ....

Describe how you felt? ....

....

Does your unique body process this food easily? ....

How did you feel today (or yesterday if you're writing this in the morning)?

....

QUOTE OF THE DAY:

66 If you were sitting on a hill in a meadow surrounded by nature and removed from any fear, you would feel good. Your natural state of being, free from the pressures and stress of your society, is one of well-being. Your natural set point is one that feels really good. You were designed to feel good. It is your birthright to feel good. Feeling good is an important part of living in physical reality. Everything you want in life is for one reason only: you think that the having of what you want will cause you to feel good." *Joshua*

MEDITATION:

Duration .... Type...

Time of Day .... Satisfaction Level: 1 2 3 4 5 6 7 8 9 10

Notes: ....

....

Appreciation: (List 5 things you appreciate about your life)

1. ....

2. ....

3. ....

4. ....

5. ....

Gratitude: (List 5 things you are grateful for, which can include future manifestations)

1. ....

2. ....

3. ....

4. ....

5. ....

Set your general intentions for the day:

....

....

....

Write five affirmations:

1. ....

2. ....

3. ....

4. ....

5. ....

How did you feel today (or yesterday if you're writing this in the morning)?

....

....

How do you feel now? ....

How do you intend to feel today (or tomorrow if you're writing this in the evening)?

....

....

INSPIRATION:

Did you receive inspiration today (or yesterday if you're writing this in the morning)?

....

....

Describe what you were inspired to do or say ....

....

FOOD EXPERIMENT:

What single item of food did you experiment with today (or yesterday if you're writing this in the morning)? ....

Describe how you felt? ....

....

Does your unique body process this food easily? ....

How did you feel today (or yesterday if you're writing this in the morning)?

....

QUOTE OF THE DAY:

66 Imagine that from this day forward you decided that the most important thing is how you felt in every moment of the day. If you were determined to feel good, how would that look? What would you do? If it was your priority in life to simply feel good, you would start with how you deal with your emotions. The only thing that ever causes you not to feel good is negative emotion. Without negative emotion, you would naturally feel good. However, you do not want to rid yourself of bad-feeling emotions because that is half of your guidance system. You simply want to manage your response to negative emotion." *Joshua*

MEDITATION:

Duration .... Type...

Time of Day .... Satisfaction Level: 1 2 3 4 5 6 7 8 9 10

Notes: ....

....

Appreciation: (List 5 things you appreciate about your life)

1. ....

2. ....

3. ....

4. ....

5. ....

Gratitude: (List 5 things you are grateful for, which can include future manifestations)

1. ....

2. ....

3. ....

4. ....

5. ....

Set your general intentions for the day:

....

....

....

Write five affirmations:

1. ....

2. ....

3. ....

4. ....

5. ....

How did you feel today (or yesterday if you're writing this in the morning)?

....

....

How do you feel now? ....

How do you intend to feel today (or tomorrow if you're writing this in the evening)?

....

....

INSPIRATION:

Did you receive inspiration today (or yesterday if you're writing this in the morning)?

....

....

Describe what you were inspired to do or say ....

....

FOOD EXPERIMENT:

What single item of food did you experiment with today (or yesterday if you're writing this in the morning)? ....

Describe how you felt? ....

....

Does your unique body process this food easily?..

How did you feel today (or yesterday if you're writing this in the morning)?

....

QUOTE OF THE DAY:

" If you could get to the point where you embraced those occasions where you felt negative emotion, and you could know that this is your opportunity to change, then negative emotion would not feel so bad. You would have a new perspective. You would see that the negative emotion is just there to guide you. It feels bad, but that's okay and it won't feel bad for long because you are quick to adopt a higher perspective that allows you to feel relief and return to feeling good." *Joshua*

MEDITATION:

Duration .... Type...

Time of Day .... Satisfaction Level: 1 2 3 4 5 6 7 8 9 10

Notes: ....

....

Appreciation: (List 5 things you appreciate about your life)

1. ....

2. ....

3. ....

4. ....

5. ....

Gratitude: (List 5 things you are grateful for, which can include future manifestations)

1. ....

2. ....

3. ....

4. ....

5. ....

Set your general intentions for the day:

....

....

....

Write five affirmations:

1. ....
2. ....
3. ....
4. ....
5. ....

How did you feel today (or yesterday if you're writing this in the morning)?

....

....

How do you feel now? ....

How do you intend to feel today (or tomorrow if you're writing this in the evening)?

....

....

INSPIRATION:

Did you receive inspiration today (or yesterday if you're writing this in the morning)?

....

....

Describe what you were inspired to do or say ....

....

FOOD EXPERIMENT:

What single item of food did you experiment with today (or yesterday if you're writing this in the morning)? ....

Describe how you felt? ....

....

Does your unique body process this food easily? ....

How did you feel today (or yesterday if you're writing this in the morning)?

....

QUOTE OF THE DAY:

" To feel good you must know that bad-feeling emotions are very good things. If you keep resisting and fighting the messages contained in your emotions, you will feel bad for longer periods of time. Imagine if you could get to a place where when someone says something hurtful, you could embrace it with love. That is true power. There is nothing more powerful than that. If you could see it for what it really is, you would easily slip off the limiting aspects of your persona and allow it to continually shift and move and change so that you could become a vibrational match to everything you ever wanted. Anything less than that is simply resistance." *Joshua*

MEDITATION:

Duration .... Type...

Time of Day .... Satisfaction Level: 1 2 3 4 5 6 7 8 9 10

Notes: ....

....

Appreciation: (List 5 things you appreciate about your life)

1. ....
2. ....
3. ....
4. ....
5. ....

Gratitude: (List 5 things you are grateful for, which can include future manifestations)

1. ....
2. ....
3. ....
4. ....
5. ....

Set your general intentions for the day:

....

....

....

Write five affirmations:

1. ....
2. ....
3. ....
4. ....
5. ....

How did you feel today (or yesterday if you're writing this in the morning)?

....

....

How do you feel now? ....

How do you intend to feel today (or tomorrow if you're writing this in the evening)?

....

....

INSPIRATION:

Did you receive inspiration today (or yesterday if you're writing this in the morning)?

....

....

Describe what you were inspired to do or say ....

....

FOOD EXPERIMENT:

What single item of food did you experiment with today (or yesterday if you're writing this in the morning)? ....

Describe how you felt? ....

....

Does your unique body process this food easily? ....

How did you feel today (or yesterday if you're writing this in the morning)?

....

DAY 69: _____ / _____ / _____   M T W T F S S

QUOTE OF THE DAY:

❝ When you worry about something, you are imagining a false reality. You are thinking about the negative potential that could happen. You are creating your own fear. Since you cannot know what will happen, you use your imagination to assume the best (hope) or the worst (worry). Your future unfolds based on your vibration, not what you think should or could happen." *Joshua*

MEDITATION:

Duration .... Type...

Time of Day .... Satisfaction Level: 1 2 3 4 5 6 7 8 9 10

Notes: ....

....

....

Appreciation: (List 5 things you appreciate about your life)

1. ....
2. ....
3. ....
4. ....
5. ....

Gratitude: (List 5 things you are grateful for, which can include future manifestations)

1. ....
2. ....
3. ....
4. ....
5. ....

Set your general intentions for the day:

....

....

....

Write five affirmations:

1. ....

2. ....

3. ....

4. ....

5. ....

How did you feel today (or yesterday if you're writing this in the morning)?

....

....

How do you feel now? ....

How do you intend to feel today (or tomorrow if you're writing this in the evening)?

....

....

INSPIRATION:

Did you receive inspiration today (or yesterday if you're writing this in the morning)?

....

....

Describe what you were inspired to do or say ....

....

FOOD EXPERIMENT:

What single item of food did you experiment with today (or yesterday if you're writing this in the morning)? ....

Describe how you felt? ....

....

Does your unique body process this food easily? ....

How did you feel today (or yesterday if you're writing this in the morning)?

....

QUOTE OF THE DAY:

" Negative emotion means that you are looking at something from a perspective that is not aligned with the person you need to become in order to receive what you want. Positive emotion means that you are looking at the subject from a perspective that is perfectly aligned with the person you are becoming who will be a match to your desire. If you have negative emotion, it means you have a desire. The stronger the negative emotion, the stronger your desire. If you feel strong negative emotion, it means that the desire is also strong and your perspective is completely different from the perspective you would have if you were a match to your desire." *Joshua*

MEDITATION:

Duration .... Type...

Time of Day .... Satisfaction Level: 1 2 3 4 5 6 7 8 9 10

Notes: ....

....

Appreciation: (List 5 things you appreciate about your life)

1. ....

2. ....

3. ....

4. ....

5. ....

Gratitude: (List 5 things you are grateful for, which can include future manifestations)

1. ....

2. ....

3. ....

4. ....

5. ....

Set your general intentions for the day:

....

....

....

Write five affirmations:

1. ....

2. ....

3. ....

4. ....

5. ....

How did you feel today (or yesterday if you're writing this in the morning)?

....

....

How do you feel now? ....

How do you intend to feel today (or tomorrow if you're writing this in the evening)?

....

....

INSPIRATION:

Did you receive inspiration today (or yesterday if you're writing this in the morning)?

....

....

Describe what you were inspired to do or say ....

....

FOOD EXPERIMENT:

What single item of food did you experiment with today (or yesterday if you're writing this in the morning)? ....

Describe how you felt? ....

....

Does your unique body process this food easily? ....

How did you feel today (or yesterday if you're writing this in the morning)?

....

QUOTE OF THE DAY:

" If you knew the magnificence that is you, you could literally be, do, and have anything you wanted. If you understood fully that you create your own reality, you would utilize the knowledge of the powers of the universe, which you have access to now, to create whatever feeling you desire in the moment. You would hold how you feel as the most important aspect of physical reality and you would strive to feel good." *Joshua*

MEDITATION:

Duration .... Type..

Time of Day .... Satisfaction Level: 1 2 3 4 5 6 7 8 9 10

Notes: ....

....

....

Appreciation: (List 5 things you appreciate about your life)

1. ....

2. ....

3. ....

4. ....

5. ....

Gratitude: (List 5 things you are grateful for, which can include future manifestations)

1. ....

2. ....

3. ....

4. ....

5. ....

Set your general intentions for the day:

....

....

....

Write five affirmations:

1. ....

2. ....

3. ....

4. ....

5. ....

How did you feel today (or yesterday if you're writing this in the morning)?

....

....

How do you feel now? ....

How do you intend to feel today (or tomorrow if you're writing this in the evening)?

....

....

INSPIRATION:

Did you receive inspiration today (or yesterday if you're writing this in the morning)?

....

....

Describe what you were inspired to do or say ....

....

FOOD EXPERIMENT:

What single item of food did you experiment with today (or yesterday if you're writing this in the morning)? ....

Describe how you felt? ....

....

Does your unique body process this food easily? ....

How did you feel today (or yesterday if you're writing this in the morning)?

....

QUOTE OF THE DAY:

" If you were to live in physical reality completely aware of who you really are, you would view nothing as wrong. You would find a perspective that would allow you to see things as right. You might not personally prefer certain things, but you would remove your attention from those things, knowing that they could be right for others. You would focus your attention on what you prefer and leave the rest alone. You would not fight against anything or make anyone wrong, including yourself. As a being of pure positive love and acceptance, you would love and accept others and yourself as you are. In fact, you would consider everything as it is in the moment as perfect." *Joshua*

MEDITATION:

Duration ....   Type..

Time of Day ....   Satisfaction Level: 1 2 3 4 5 6 7 8 9 10

Notes: ....

....

Appreciation: (List 5 things you appreciate about your life)

1. ....

2. ....

3. ....

4. ....

5. ....

Gratitude: (List 5 things you are grateful for, which can include future manifestations)

1. ....

2. ....

3. ....

4. ....

5. ....

Set your general intentions for the day:

....

....

....

Write five affirmations:

1. ....

2. ....

3. ....

4. ....

5. ....

How did you feel today (or yesterday if you're writing this in the morning)?

....

....

How do you feel now? ....

How do you intend to feel today (or tomorrow if you're writing this in the evening)?

....

....

INSPIRATION:

Did you receive inspiration today (or yesterday if you're writing this in the morning)?

....

....

Describe what you were inspired to do or say ....

....

FOOD EXPERIMENT:

What single item of food did you experiment with today (or yesterday if you're writing this in the morning)? ....

Describe how you felt? ....

....

Does your unique body process this food easily?..

How did you feel today (or yesterday if you're writing this in the morning)?

....

QUOTE OF THE DAY:

" Living as who you really are would be living as an allower would live. You would not force things or struggle to push your way through; you would allow everything you want to come to you. You would become a receiver and not a doer. You know that this universe is set up to provide you with all that you want and that the only way something does not come to you is if you resist it. You know that change is not only good, but necessary and inevitable. You are constantly changing. There is no need to resist change. Change allows you to receive that which you want." *Joshua*

MEDITATION:

Duration .... Type...

Time of Day .... Satisfaction Level: 1 2 3 4 5 6 7 8 9 10

Notes: ....

....

Appreciation: (List 5 things you appreciate about your life)

1. ....

2. ....

3. ....

4. ....

5. ....

Gratitude: (List 5 things you are grateful for, which can include future manifestations)

1. ....

2. ....

3. ....

4. ....

5. ....

Set your general intentions for the day:

....

....

....

Write five affirmations:

1. ....

2. ....

3. ....

4. ....

5. ....

How did you feel today (or yesterday if you're writing this in the morning)?

....

....

How do you feel now? ....

How do you intend to feel today (or tomorrow if you're writing this in the evening)?

....

....

INSPIRATION:

Did you receive inspiration today (or yesterday if you're writing this in the morning)?

....

....

Describe what you were inspired to do or say ....

....

FOOD EXPERIMENT:

What single item of food did you experiment with today (or yesterday if you're writing this in the morning)? ....

Describe how you felt? ....

....

Does your unique body process this food easily? ....

How did you feel today (or yesterday if you're writing this in the morning)?

....

DAY 74: _____ / _____ / _____   M T W T F S S

QUOTE OF THE DAY:

" Nothing is wrong. Everything is right. If you can live by this one statement, your life will get easier. A life of ease allows all that you want to come. Create ease in your life by starting to see how everything could be right. When your mate does something you do not like, instead of making them wrong, see how they could be right. You can't change anyone, even if you think you can. You are simply causing them to temporarily modify their behavior. When you ask them to be someone they are not, you are trying to change the conditions outside of you and this creates conflict and stress. Instead, change yourself." *Joshua*

MEDITATION:

Duration .... Type..

Time of Day .... Satisfaction Level: 1 2 3 4 5 6 7 8 9 10

Notes: ....

....

Appreciation: (List 5 things you appreciate about your life)

1. ....
2. ....
3. ....
4. ....
5. ....

Gratitude: (List 5 things you are grateful for, which can include future manifestations)

1. ....
2. ....
3. ....
4. ....
5. ....

Set your general intentions for the day:

....

....

....

Write five affirmations:

1. ....

2. ....

3. ....

4. ....

5. ....

How did you feel today (or yesterday if you're writing this in the morning)?

....

....

How do you feel now? ....

How do you intend to feel today (or tomorrow if you're writing this in the evening)?

....

....

INSPIRATION:

Did you receive inspiration today (or yesterday if you're writing this in the morning)?

....

....

Describe what you were inspired to do or say ....

....

FOOD EXPERIMENT:

What single item of food did you experiment with today (or yesterday if you're writing this in the morning)? ....

Describe how you felt? ....

....

Does your unique body process this food easily? ....

How did you feel today (or yesterday if you're writing this in the morning)?

....

QUOTE OF THE DAY:

" Everything happens for you. If your mate does something you do not like, they did it specifically for you. That's how it is right. They are challenging your belief system. They are letting you peek into a limiting belief that is based in some irrational fear. Look at the fear rather than asking them not to do things that cause you to feel fear." *Joshua*

MEDITATION:

Duration .... Type..

Time of Day .... Satisfaction Level: 1 2 3 4 5 6 7 8 9 10

Notes: ....

....

Appreciation: (List 5 things you appreciate about your life)

1. ....

2. ....

3. ....

4. ....

5. ....

Gratitude: (List 5 things you are grateful for, which can include future manifestations)

1. ....

2. ....

3. ....

4. ....

5. ....

Set your general intentions for the day:

....

....

....

....

Write five affirmations:

1. ....

2. ....

3. ....

4. ....

5. ....

How did you feel today (or yesterday if you're writing this in the morning)?

....

....

How do you feel now? ....

How do you intend to feel today (or tomorrow if you're writing this in the evening)?

....

....

INSPIRATION:

Did you receive inspiration today (or yesterday if you're writing this in the morning)?

....

....

Describe what you were inspired to do or say ....

....

FOOD EXPERIMENT:

What single item of food did you experiment with today (or yesterday if you're writing this in the morning)? ....

Describe how you felt? ....

....

Does your unique body process this food easily? ....

How did you feel today (or yesterday if you're writing this in the morning)?

....

QUOTE OF THE DAY:

" Everything is right. If it is happening, it is happening for you no matter what it is. If you are aware of it, then it is for you. If you are not aware of it, then it is not for you. That's how you can tell. If someone says something nice to you, then that is for your benefit and growth. It reinforces a beneficial belief. If someone says something rude to you, then that is for your benefit, because it allows you to take a look at a limiting belief you have about yourself. It is always, always for you." *Joshua*

MEDITATION:

Duration .... Type..

Time of Day .... Satisfaction Level: 1 2 3 4 5 6 7 8 9 10

Notes: ....

....

Appreciation: (List 5 things you appreciate about your life)

1. ....

2. ....

3. ....

4. ....

5. ....

Gratitude: (List 5 things you are grateful for, which can include future manifestations)

1. ....

2. ....

3. ....

4. ....

5. ....

Set your general intentions for the day:

....

....

....

Write five affirmations:

1. ....
2. ....
3. ....
4. ....
5. ....

How did you feel today (or yesterday if you're writing this in the morning)?

....

....

How do you feel now? ....

How do you intend to feel today (or tomorrow if you're writing this in the evening)?

....

....

INSPIRATION:

Did you receive inspiration today (or yesterday if you're writing this in the morning)?

....

....

Describe what you were inspired to do or say ....

....

FOOD EXPERIMENT:

What single item of food did you experiment with today (or yesterday if you're writing this in the morning)? ....

Describe how you felt? ....

....

Does your unique body process this food easily?..

How did you feel today (or yesterday if you're writing this in the morning)?

....

QUOTE OF THE DAY:

❝ Everything is right for someone, somewhere. If it is not something you prefer, that's okay. Just remove your attention from it. It is not your place to decide what is good or bad, right or wrong for anyone else. They all came here to explore reality in their own way and they are all expanding as a result. Just because you cannot see the benefit of a life they chose doesn't mean that it is not a valid way to explore physical reality." *Joshua*

MEDITATION:

Duration .... Type...

Time of Day .... Satisfaction Level: 1 2 3 4 5 6 7 8 9 10

Notes: ....

....

Appreciation: (List 5 things you appreciate about your life)

1. ....

2. ....

3. ....

4. ....

5. ....

Gratitude: (List 5 things you are grateful for, which can include future manifestations)

1. ....

2. ....

3. ....

4. ....

5. ....

Set your general intentions for the day:

....

....

....

....

Write five affirmations:

1. ....
2. ....
3. ....
4. ....
5. ....

How did you feel today (or yesterday if you're writing this in the morning)?

....

....

How do you feel now? ....

How do you intend to feel today (or tomorrow if you're writing this in the evening)?

....

....

INSPIRATION:

Did you receive inspiration today (or yesterday if you're writing this in the morning)?

....

....

Describe what you were inspired to do or say ....

....

FOOD EXPERIMENT:

What single item of food did you experiment with today (or yesterday if you're writing this in the morning)? ....

Describe how you felt? ....

....

Does your unique body process this food easily? ....

How did you feel today (or yesterday if you're writing this in the morning)?

....

QUOTE OF THE DAY:

" From your perspective you cannot see how some things might be right and that's okay. There are a lot of things going on in this world. That is by design. There have never been more people on the planet. That is because there has never been such diversity and opportunities for exploration. More are coming now because frankly there's a whole lot more to explore." *Joshua*

MEDITATION:

Duration ....   Type...

Time of Day ....   Satisfaction Level: 1 2 3 4 5 6 7 8 9 10

Notes: ....

....

Appreciation: (List 5 things you appreciate about your life)

1. ....

2. ....

3. ....

4. ....

5. ....

Gratitude: (List 5 things you are grateful for, which can include future manifestations)

1. ....

2. ....

3. ....

4. ....

5. ....

Set your general intentions for the day:

....

....

....

....

Write five affirmations:

1. ....

2. ....

3. ....

4. ....

5. ....

How did you feel today (or yesterday if you're writing this in the morning)?

....

....

How do you feel now? ....

How do you intend to feel today (or tomorrow if you're writing this in the evening)?

....

....

INSPIRATION:

Did you receive inspiration today (or yesterday if you're writing this in the morning)?

....

....

Describe what you were inspired to do or say ....

....

FOOD EXPERIMENT:

What single item of food did you experiment with today (or yesterday if you're writing this in the morning)? ....

Describe how you felt? ....

....

Does your unique body process this food easily? ....

How did you feel today (or yesterday if you're writing this in the morning)?

....

QUOTE OF THE DAY:

" You are a limitless being of pure positive love and acceptance. To be loving is to be accepting. To accept others as they are means that you must first accept yourself as you are. You must accept yourself with all your qualities, some of which you judge as good and some you judge as bad. What are your good qualities? List them now. Take out a pen and paper and in your own hand write a list of your top twenty best qualities. Are you smart? Are you funny? Are you loyal? Are you giving? Are you talented in some area? Do you have good taste? Do you like animals? Can you see beauty? Are you creative?" *Joshua*

MEDITATION:

Duration .... Type ....

Time of Day .... Satisfaction Level: 1 2 3 4 5 6 7 8 9 10

Notes: ....

....

Appreciation: (List 5 things you appreciate about your life)

1. ....

2. ....

3. ....

4. ....

5. ....

Gratitude: (List 5 things you are grateful for, which can include future manifestations)

1. ....

2. ....

3. ....

4. ....

5. ....

Set your general intentions for the day:

....

....

....

Write five affirmations:

1. ....

2. ....

3. ....

4. ....

5. ....

How did you feel today (or yesterday if you're writing this in the morning)?

....

....

How do you feel now? ....

How do you intend to feel today (or tomorrow if you're writing this in the evening)?

....

....

INSPIRATION:

Did you receive inspiration today (or yesterday if you're writing this in the morning)?

....

....

Describe what you were inspired to do or say ....

....

FOOD EXPERIMENT:

What single item of food did you experiment with today (or yesterday if you're writing this in the morning)? ....

Describe how you felt? ....

....

Does your unique body process this food easily? ....

How did you feel today (or yesterday if you're writing this in the morning)?

....

QUOTE OF THE DAY:

" When you act out of love rather than fear, you allow the universe to do the work for you. Your limiting beliefs are limiting what the universe can bring. Start thinking in a limitless way. Start thinking bigger. Start imagining that nothing can go wrong, for that is entirely accurate. If something goes wrong, it's simply pointing out another limiting belief. Don't worry, move ahead and be captivated by what unfolds. It is all within your power when you view yourself as a limitless being of pure positive love and acceptance." *Joshua*

MEDITATION:

Duration .... Type..

Time of Day .... Satisfaction Level: 1 2 3 4 5 6 7 8 9 10

Notes: ....

....

Appreciation: (List 5 things you appreciate about your life)

   1. ....

   2. ....

   3. ....

   4. ....

   5. ....

Gratitude: (List 5 things you are grateful for, which can include future manifestations)

   1. ....

   2. ....

   3. ....

   4. ....

   5. ....

Set your general intentions for the day:

....

....

....

Write five affirmations:

1. ....

2. ....

3. ....

4. ....

5. ....

How did you feel today (or yesterday if you're writing this in the morning)?

....

....

How do you feel now? ....

How do you intend to feel today (or tomorrow if you're writing this in the evening)?

....

....

INSPIRATION:

Did you receive inspiration today (or yesterday if you're writing this in the morning)?

....

....

Describe what you were inspired to do or say ....

....

FOOD EXPERIMENT:

What single item of food did you experiment with today (or yesterday if you're writing this in the morning)? ....

Describe how you felt? ....

....

Does your unique body process this food easily? ....

How did you feel today (or yesterday if you're writing this in the morning)?

....

QUOTE OF THE DAY:

" A self-directed life is one where you place yourself first. We will tell you that physical reality is an illusion. It is a very convincing illusion. You believe you are one of several billion people living on this planet. You think you are an individual drop of water in a vast sea. You believe that you are not that important or special. But there is a secret. The secret is this: you are the center of your universe." *Joshua*

MEDITATION:

Duration .... Type..

Time of Day .... Satisfaction Level: 1 2 3 4 5 6 7 8 9 10

Notes: ....

....

Appreciation: (List 5 things you appreciate about your life)

1. ....

2. ....

3. ....

4. ....

5. ....

Gratitude: (List 5 things you are grateful for, which can include future manifestations)

1. ....

2. ....

3. ....

4. ....

5. ....

Set your general intentions for the day:

....

....

....

....

Write five affirmations:

1. ....

2. ....

3. ....

4. ....

5. ....

How did you feel today (or yesterday if you're writing this in the morning)?

....

....

How do you feel now? ....

How do you intend to feel today (or tomorrow if you're writing this in the evening)?

....

....

INSPIRATION:

Did you receive inspiration today (or yesterday if you're writing this in the morning)?

....

....

Describe what you were inspired to do or say ....

....

FOOD EXPERIMENT:

What single item of food did you experiment with today (or yesterday if you're writing this in the morning)? ....

Describe how you felt? ....

....

Does your unique body process this food easily? ....

How did you feel today (or yesterday if you're writing this in the morning)?

....

QUOTE OF THE DAY:

" The reason you do not allow what you want to come to you is because you believe in right and wrong. For you personally, there are right ways to do things and there are wrong ways to do things. Some things are good and some things are bad. You judge this method for receiving what you want as good and this other method as bad. That's all fine; however, based on the beliefs you've adopted from others, it's limiting." *Joshua*

MEDITATION:

Duration .... Type..

Time of Day .... Satisfaction Level: 1 2 3 4 5 6 7 8 9 10

Notes: ....

....

Appreciation: (List 5 things you appreciate about your life)

1. ....

2. ....

3. ....

4. ....

5. ....

Gratitude: (List 5 things you are grateful for, which can include future manifestations)

1. ....

2. ....

3. ....

4. ....

5. ....

Set your general intentions for the day:

....

....

....

....

Write five affirmations:

1. ....

2. ....

3. ....

4. ....

5. ....

How did you feel today (or yesterday if you're writing this in the morning)?

....

....

How do you feel now? ....

How do you intend to feel today (or tomorrow if you're writing this in the evening)?

....

....

INSPIRATION:

Did you receive inspiration today (or yesterday if you're writing this in the morning)?

....

....

Describe what you were inspired to do or say ....

....

FOOD EXPERIMENT:

What single item of food did you experiment with today (or yesterday if you're writing this in the morning)? ....

Describe how you felt? ....

....

Does your unique body process this food easily? ....

How did you feel today (or yesterday if you're writing this in the morning)?

....

QUOTE OF THE DAY:

66 There is nothing wrong with living a limited life. That's how the vast majority of people operate. They are held prisoner by their own belief system. The tragedy is that most of your beliefs were adopted from others who had those same beliefs. You did not have the actual experience; you just listened to an old story and picked up the belief the same way you pick up a virus. Your body has defenses against a virus. We have shown you how to defend against a limiting belief. The question is whether you will do the work or not." *Joshua*

MEDITATION:

Duration .... Type..

Time of Day .... Satisfaction Level: 1 2 3 4 5 6 7 8 9 10

Notes: ....

....

Appreciation: (List 5 things you appreciate about your life)

1. ....

2. ....

3. ....

4. ....

5. ....

Gratitude: (List 5 things you are grateful for, which can include future manifestations)

1. ....

2. ....

3. ....

4. ....

5. ....

Set your general intentions for the day:

....

....

....

Write five affirmations:

1. ....

2. ....

3. ....

4. ....

5. ....

How did you feel today (or yesterday if you're writing this in the morning)?

....

....

How do you feel now? ....

How do you intend to feel today (or tomorrow if you're writing this in the evening)?

....

....

INSPIRATION:

Did you receive inspiration today (or yesterday if you're writing this in the morning)?

....

....

Describe what you were inspired to do or say ....

....

FOOD EXPERIMENT:

What single item of food did you experiment with today (or yesterday if you're writing this in the morning)? ....

Describe how you felt? ....

....

Does your unique body process this food easily? ....

How did you feel today (or yesterday if you're writing this in the morning)?

....

QUOTE OF THE DAY:

" Everything you want is coming to you if you will just allow it. How do you allow what you want to come? You reduce your resistance. How do you reduce resistance? You believe that nothing is wrong or bad. If you believe something is wrong, you have just resisted it. If you think something is bad, you have just resisted it." *Joshua*

MEDITATION:

Duration .... Type...

Time of Day .... Satisfaction Level: 1 2 3 4 5 6 7 8 9 10

Notes: ....

....

....

Appreciation: (List 5 things you appreciate about your life)

1. ....

2. ....

3. ....

4. ....

5. ....

Gratitude: (List 5 things you are grateful for, which can include future manifestations)

1. ....

2. ....

3. ....

4. ....

5. ....

Set your general intentions for the day:

....

....

....

....

Write five affirmations:

1. ....
2. ....
3. ....
4. ....
5. ....

How did you feel today (or yesterday if you're writing this in the morning)?

....

....

How do you feel now? ....

How do you intend to feel today (or tomorrow if you're writing this in the evening)?

....

....

INSPIRATION:

Did you receive inspiration today (or yesterday if you're writing this in the morning)?

....

....

Describe what you were inspired to do or say ....

....

FOOD EXPERIMENT:

What single item of food did you experiment with today (or yesterday if you're writing this in the morning)? ....

Describe how you felt? ....

....

Does your unique body process this food easily? ....

How did you feel today (or yesterday if you're writing this in the morning)?

....

QUOTE OF THE DAY:

" Nothing is good or bad; it is all neutral. Your habit of judgment causes you to see good things as bad and right things as wrong. This is why you personally cannot get what you want. This is why you feel stress. This is the cause of everything unwanted. This is the simple truth of physical reality." *Joshua*

MEDITATION:

Duration .... Type...

Time of Day .... Satisfaction Level: 1 2 3 4 5 6 7 8 9 10

Notes: ....

....

....

Appreciation: (List 5 things you appreciate about your life)

1. ....

2. ....

3. ....

4. ....

5. ....

Gratitude: (List 5 things you are grateful for, which can include future manifestations)

1. ....

2. ....

3. ....

4. ....

5. ....

Set your general intentions for the day:

....

....

....

....

Write five affirmations:

1. ....

2. ....

3. ....

4. ....

5. ....

How did you feel today (or yesterday if you're writing this in the morning)?

....

....

How do you feel now? ....

How do you intend to feel today (or tomorrow if you're writing this in the evening)?

....

....

INSPIRATION:

Did you receive inspiration today (or yesterday if you're writing this in the morning)?

....

....

Describe what you were inspired to do or say ....

....

FOOD EXPERIMENT:

What single item of food did you experiment with today (or yesterday if you're writing this in the morning)? ....

Describe how you felt? ....

....

Does your unique body process this food easily? ....

How did you feel today (or yesterday if you're writing this in the morning)?

....

QUOTE OF THE DAY:

❝ In an attractive reality such as this, non-resistance is the key to operating within the design of the system. All of the great successes in life come from working with the system rather than fighting against it. Some may enjoy the fight because it gives them a feeling of purpose, but the fight cannot give you what you really want. Nothing is wrong; it is always right. Things are perfect as they are now and improving with every new moment. Work within the system and you become an allower. Everything you personally want will flow to you while in the state of allowing." *Joshua*

MEDITATION:

Duration .... Type...

Time of Day .... Satisfaction Level: 1 2 3 4 5 6 7 8 9 10

Notes: ....

....

Appreciation: (List 5 things you appreciate about your life)

1. ....

2. ....

3. ....

4. ....

5. ....

Gratitude: (List 5 things you are grateful for, which can include future manifestations)

1. ....

2. ....

3. ....

4. ....

5. ....

Set your general intentions for the day:

....

....

....

Write five affirmations:

1. ....

2. ....

3. ....

4. ....

5. ....

How did you feel today (or yesterday if you're writing this in the morning)?

....

....

How do you feel now? ....

How do you intend to feel today (or tomorrow if you're writing this in the evening)?

....

....

INSPIRATION:

Did you receive inspiration today (or yesterday if you're writing this in the morning)?

....

....

Describe what you were inspired to do or say ....

....

FOOD EXPERIMENT:

What single item of food did you experiment with today (or yesterday if you're writing this in the morning)? ....

Describe how you felt? ....

....

Does your unique body process this food easily? ....

How did you feel today (or yesterday if you're writing this in the morning)?

....

QUOTE OF THE DAY:

❝ You can look at anything and feel good. You can use anything as your excuse to feel good. You can choose to enjoy life and feel good. You can also look at the things you lack and feel bad. You can look at the lives of others and by comparison you can feel bad. Feeling bad is easy. You've been doing it for a long time. However, unless you purposely choose to feel good, you will not change your life in a meaningful way. From now on you will do the work required to feel good." *Joshua*

MEDITATION:

Duration .... Type...

Time of Day .... Satisfaction Level: 1 2 3 4 5 6 7 8 9 10

Notes: ....

....

Appreciation: (List 5 things you appreciate about your life)

1. ....

2. ....

3. ....

4. ....

5. ....

Gratitude: (List 5 things you are grateful for, which can include future manifestations)

1. ....

2. ....

3. ....

4. ....

5. ....

Set your general intentions for the day:

....

....

....

Write five affirmations:

1. ....

2. ....

3. ....

4. ....

5. ....

How did you feel today (or yesterday if you're writing this in the morning)?

....

....

How do you feel now? ....

How do you intend to feel today (or tomorrow if you're writing this in the evening)?

....

....

INSPIRATION:

Did you receive inspiration today (or yesterday if you're writing this in the morning)?

....

....

Describe what you were inspired to do or say ....

....

FOOD EXPERIMENT:

What single item of food did you experiment with today (or yesterday if you're writing this in the morning)? ....

Describe how you felt? ....

....

Does your unique body process this food easily?...

How did you feel today (or yesterday if you're writing this in the morning)?

....

QUOTE OF THE DAY:

❝ Nothing is wrong, so there's no need to complain. There's no purpose in talking about what you do not like. This is your habit and it's contradictory. The universe does not understand that you don't like something, but for some reason you enjoy talking about it. It doesn't make sense given the fundamental design of the system. Why would you put your attention on anything you don't like when your attention is the tool for bringing you more of whatever you are focused on? If you focus on something you do not like by talking about it, then all you are doing is asking the universe to bring you more of it. If you do not like it, if you think it's bad or wrong, don't talk about it; instead, find a way to see it as right or remove your attention from it." *Joshua*

MEDITATION:

Duration .... Type..

Time of Day .... Satisfaction Level: 1 2 3 4 5 6 7 8 9 10

Notes: ....

....

Appreciation: (List 5 things you appreciate about your life)

1. ....

2. ....

3. ....

4. ....

5. ....

Gratitude: (List 5 things you are grateful for, which can include future manifestations)

1. ....

2. ....

3. ....

4. ....

5. ....

Set your general intentions for the day:

....

....

Write five affirmations:

1. ....

2. ....

3. ....

4. ....

5. ....

How did you feel today (or yesterday if you're writing this in the morning)?

....

....

How do you feel now? ....

How do you intend to feel today (or tomorrow if you're writing this in the evening)?

....

....

INSPIRATION:

Did you receive inspiration today (or yesterday if you're writing this in the morning)?

....

....

Describe what you were inspired to do or say ....

....

FOOD EXPERIMENT:

What single item of food did you experiment with today (or yesterday if you're writing this in the morning)? ....

Describe how you felt? ....

....

Does your unique body process this food easily? ....

How did you feel today (or yesterday if you're writing this in the morning)?

....

QUOTE OF THE DAY:

❝ Simply by refraining from complaining and instead working to see it in a positive light, your life will shift upwards so dramatically that you won't truly believe it. You might not believe that such a simple change in your approach to life could cause such a profound shift in your reality. But it is true. You see, by refusing to complain and then choosing to see the beauty in the ugly, you change your entire point of attraction. You raise your vibration from low to high with one simple change in your approach. You move from fighting against the system of reality to engaging the leverage of universal forces. You go from paddling upstream to floating downstream. It's as simple as that." *Joshua*

MEDITATION:

Duration .... Type..

Time of Day .... Satisfaction Level: 1 2 3 4 5 6 7 8 9 10

Notes: ....

....

Appreciation: (List 5 things you appreciate about your life)

1. ....

2. ....

3. ....

4. ....

5. ....

Gratitude: (List 5 things you are grateful for, which can include future manifestations)

1. ....

2. ....

3. ....

4. ....

5. ....

Set your general intentions for the day:

....

....

....

Write five affirmations:

1. ....

2. ....

3. ....

4. ....

5. ....

How did you feel today (or yesterday if you're writing this in the morning)?

....

....

How do you feel now? ....

How do you intend to feel today (or tomorrow if you're writing this in the evening)?

....

....

INSPIRATION:

Did you receive inspiration today (or yesterday if you're writing this in the morning)?

....

....

Describe what you were inspired to do or say ....

....

FOOD EXPERIMENT:

What single item of food did you experiment with today (or yesterday if you're writing this in the morning)? ....

Describe how you felt? ....

....

Does your unique body process this food easily? ....

How did you feel today (or yesterday if you're writing this in the morning)?

....

QUOTE OF THE DAY:

❝ Stress is caused by an uncontrolled mind. When you imagine unpleasant future conditions, you create stress. It is fear. It is focus on what's not wanted. You can choose any thought. You can choose to imagine your future without what you want or with what you want. You can worry about this and that, but the future is an illusion. The only thing that matters is how you feel now in this present moment." *Joshua*

MEDITATION:

Duration .... Type...

Time of Day .... Satisfaction Level: 1 2 3 4 5 6 7 8 9 10

Notes: ....

....

....

Appreciation: (List 5 things you appreciate about your life)

1. ....

2. ....

3. ....

4. ....

5. ....

Gratitude: (List 5 things you are grateful for, which can include future manifestations)

1. ....

2. ....

3. ....

4. ....

5. ....

Set your general intentions for the day:

....

....

....

Write five affirmations:

1. ....

2. ....

3. ....

4. ....

5. ....

How did you feel today (or yesterday if you're writing this in the morning)?

....

....

How do you feel now? ....

How do you intend to feel today (or tomorrow if you're writing this in the evening)?

....

....

INSPIRATION:

Did you receive inspiration today (or yesterday if you're writing this in the morning)?

....

....

Describe what you were inspired to do or say ....

....

FOOD EXPERIMENT:

What single item of food did you experiment with today (or yesterday if you're writing this in the morning)? ....

Describe how you felt? ....

....

Does your unique body process this food easily? ....

How did you feel today (or yesterday if you're writing this in the morning)?

....

QUOTE OF THE DAY:

66 Inner conflict occurs when you believe that something bad is occurring in the moment. Stress occurs when you believe that something bad will happen in the future. Relieve your inner conflict by realizing that everything is happening for you. Relieve your stress by understanding that everything is always working out for you. If you can come to this realization, you will experience far less inner conflict and stress." *Joshua*

MEDITATION:

Duration .... Type..

Time of Day .... Satisfaction Level: 1   2   3   4   5   6   7   8   9   10

Notes: ....

....

Appreciation: (List 5 things you appreciate about your life)

1. ....

2. ....

3. ....

4. ....

5. ....

Gratitude: (List 5 things you are grateful for, which can include future manifestations)

1. ....

2. ....

3. ....

4. ....

5. ....

Set your general intentions for the day:

....

....

....

....

Write five affirmations:

1. ....

2. ....

3. ....

4. ....

5. ....

How did you feel today (or yesterday if you're writing this in the morning)?

....

....

How do you feel now? ....

How do you intend to feel today (or tomorrow if you're writing this in the evening)?

....

....

INSPIRATION:

Did you receive inspiration today (or yesterday if you're writing this in the morning)?

....

....

Describe what you were inspired to do or say ....

....

FOOD EXPERIMENT:

What single item of food did you experiment with today (or yesterday if you're writing this in the morning)? ....

Describe how you felt? ....

....

Does your unique body process this food easily? ....

How did you feel today (or yesterday if you're writing this in the morning)?

....

QUOTE OF THE DAY:

" The realization that you are taken care of, that everything is happening for you, and that everything is always working out for you will give you ease. Ease creates an environment of allowing. In this environment, where you have little stress, where you understand that there is nothing to worry about, where you are able to know the purpose of your emotions, where you are not trying to change the conditions in the moment, where you are focused on what it is you really want, you become an allower. Everything you want flows to you in this state. In the allowing state there is little resistance. Whenever a little resistance shows itself by way of some negative emotion, you react by going inside, finding the fear, and practicing the art of analysis." *Joshua*

MEDITATION:

Duration .... Type...

Time of Day .... Satisfaction Level: 1 2 3 4 5 6 7 8 9 10

Notes: ....

....

Appreciation: (List 5 things you appreciate about your life)

  1. ....

  2. ....

  3. ....

  4. ....

  5. ....

Gratitude: (List 5 things you are grateful for, which can include future manifestations)

  1. ....

  2. ....

  3. ....

  4. ....

  5. ....

Set your general intentions for the day:

....

....

Write five affirmations:

1. ....
2. ....
3. ....
4. ....
5. ....

How did you feel today (or yesterday if you're writing this in the morning)?

....

....

How do you feel now? ....

How do you intend to feel today (or tomorrow if you're writing this in the evening)?

....

....

INSPIRATION:

Did you receive inspiration today (or yesterday if you're writing this in the morning)?

....

....

Describe what you were inspired to do or say ....

....

FOOD EXPERIMENT:

What single item of food did you experiment with today (or yesterday if you're writing this in the morning)? ....

Describe how you felt? ....

....

Does your unique body process this food easily? ....

How did you feel today (or yesterday if you're writing this in the morning)?

....

QUOTE OF THE DAY:

❝ Now it is time to control your mind. Now it is time to free your mind. Now it is time to demand that you feel good. Now it is finally time to think of yourself. This is your universe and everything revolves around you. You must begin to start thinking in a way that empowers you. You must begin to think fearlessly. You must pay a little more attention to the thoughts you chronically think. You must work to free yourself of your limiting beliefs. This is the only thing you need to do. Nothing else really matters. When you begin to place how you feel above all else, everything else will magically move into place." *Joshua*

MEDITATION:

Duration .... Type..

Time of Day .... Satisfaction Level: 1 2 3 4 5 6 7 8 9 10

Notes: ....

....

Appreciation: (List 5 things you appreciate about your life)

1. ....

2. ....

3. ....

4. ....

5. ....

Gratitude: (List 5 things you are grateful for, which can include future manifestations)

1. ....

2. ....

3. ....

4. ....

5. ....

Set your general intentions for the day:

....

....

....

Write five affirmations:

1. ....
2. ....
3. ....
4. ....
5. ....

How did you feel today (or yesterday if you're writing this in the morning)?

....

....

How do you feel now? ....

How do you intend to feel today (or tomorrow if you're writing this in the evening)?

....

....

INSPIRATION:

Did you receive inspiration today (or yesterday if you're writing this in the morning)?

....

....

Describe what you were inspired to do or say ....

....

FOOD EXPERIMENT:

What single item of food did you experiment with today (or yesterday if you're writing this in the morning)? ....

Describe how you felt? ....

....

Does your unique body process this food easily? ....

How did you feel today (or yesterday if you're writing this in the morning)?

....

Made in the USA
Charleston, SC
30 December 2016